How To Absolutely, Positively

LOOK 5 *TO* 10 YEARS YOUNGER

How To Absolutely, Positively

Look
5 *To* 10 Years
Younger

By Sharon Boyd

Printed in the United States of America.
First Printing: February 1995
Valley of the Sun Publishing, Box 38, Malibu, CA 90265

ISBN: 0-87554-584-X
Library of Congress Card Number: 94-062103

The intent of this book is to offer information to assist you in the goal of looking and feeling younger. Nothing in this book is intended to constitute or replace medical treatment, or to directly or indirectly dispense medical advice. Before making any changes in your diet or exercise program, consult your physician. If you have a pre-existing medical condition, it is essential that you consult your physician before following any of the recommendations in this book.

Contents

The Face of Aging

The Constitution of the United States of America guarantees us the rights of life, liberty and the pursuit of happiness. Nowhere is a word said about youthfulness. Yet after a certain age, for many, happiness is synonymous with youthful looks. Ponce de Leon searched for the fountain of youth; Cleopatra bathed in milk (not a bad idea—certain milk proteins help keep the skin smooth); and movie icon Humphrey Bogart coined the youth-cult phrase "Live fast, die young and leave a good-looking corpse." But you don't have to die young to remain good-looking as you realize your potential for an extended, productive life.

There are lots of theories on what causes aging: the wear-and-tear theory, the rate-of-living theory, free-radicals and cross-linking theories, defective cell enzymes and accumulated cell toxins, collagen reduction, glycosolation, slowing metabolic rates, genetic programming, and so on. Scientific journals are filled with page after page of scientists' findings on these and many other theories. It may be that aging is the result of any one or even all of these factors.

Everyone is interested in preventing or slowing down the aging process—after all, whether you believe in reincarnation or not, let's face facts: this is the only life you'll enjoy in this body, so why not enjoy the advantages of being as youthful as possible for as long as you can? Who doesn't appreciate an admiring glance?

From about the age of 25 on, the human body begins to exhibit subtle changes known as the aging process. Chronologically, everyone ages at the same rate but our subjective experience shows that not everyone *looks* the same at the same age. Some people are youthful and vigorous at 75 while others seem old at 50. Studies show that people exhibiting signs of premature aging feel a marked lack of self-confidence. When we look good, we feel good—about ourselves and the world around us. Looking as young as you feel is a vital part of being a vital person.

You won't find a scientific treatise on the theories of aging in this book—since everyone experiences the aging process, we all know what the effects are. Instead, what you'll find are hundreds of ways you can look younger—not merely tricks designed to fool the eye and provide the illusion of youth and beauty but tried-and-true techniques as well as the latest intelligence on becoming more youthful, vigorous and alive. Some of these tools not only slow the aging process but can actually assist in reversing it. The result: not only can we live longer, healthier, more productive lives, but we can look our best at the same time!

At the beginning of the twentieth century, people who lived beyond 50 were considered old. The average life expectancy in the United States was 45 years; the most common causes of death were infectious diseases and accidents. As we approach the end of this century, scientific advances in the treatment of disease have added an astonishing thirty or more years to that figure for women, slightly less for men. The current leading causes of death—cancer and heart disease—are degenerative diseases, which many researchers say to a great extent are brought on by our modern, stressful lifestyles. According to research done by the Rockefeller Foundation, over 95 percent of the people born in the world are born healthy. We age and die prematurely from our own bad habits: drugs, excessive alcohol intake, smoking, overeating, lack of exercise, inadequate sleep.

Science has made amazing breakthroughs in extending our lives, but only we can determine the quality of those additional years. As yet, there is no single formula or magic bullet that can reset your body's biological clock, but there are things you *can* do *now* to rejuvenate and re-energize yourself. You can look and feel five to ten years younger, more beautiful and full of vitality by integrating your total being—body, mind and spirit—to fight the basic aging process in your body.

Here's looking at you, kid.

REJUVENATING THE OUTER YOU

Outer Appearances

In the introduction, we promised you that you could look five to ten years younger by integrating your body, mind and spirit. This section deals with the part of your being most readily apparent to you and everyone around you—your outer appearance. We'll cover the effects of proper skin and hair care, adequate exercise, and optimal diet and nutrition on your appearance. Many bodily changes blamed on the aging process are really the result of abuse and neglect. Education and prevention—awareness and action—can remedy many of the physical signs of aging.

You will not find information about facial rejuvenation surgery—surgical nips and tucks, collagen injections, cheek implants, dermabrasion, chemical peels, or laser lifts. Those actions are beyond the scope of this book, whose main theme is practical solutions *you* can do for *yourself*. If you feel you need these aids, see your dermatologist or plastic surgeon.

Skin

...

"It is increasingly apparent that appearance, certainly including cutaneous appearance, contributes to society's evaluation of an individual's competence and to that individual's sense of self-worth and well-being. ... the prospect of effective anti-aging product for the skin may have direct medical benefit beyond its effect on premalignant lesions."—**Journal of the American Medical Association, Vol. 259, No. 4, p. 569.**

We all know the importance of first impressions. This chapter will give you all the information, tips and tools you need to put your best face forward and make that great first impression (and second, and third ...).

If you're like most people, you think the first sign of aging is wrinkled, sagging skin (grey hair runs a close second). Eliminating or diminishing wrinkles for a smooth, unlined complexion is the Holy Grail of the babyboomer generation. But before we tell you what specific actions to take to get that youthful complexion, there are some factors that are important to know first. Biologically, here's what happens to your skin as you age:

- Skin loses elasticity

- Skin loses 50 percent of the immune cells that protect against skin cancer

- Skin texture becomes rougher

- Skin loses 10 to 20 percent of its pigment cells each decade

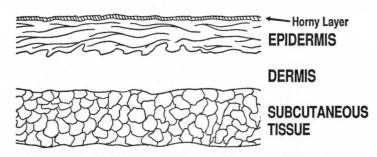

← Horny Layer
EPIDERMIS

DERMIS

SUBCUTANEOUS TISSUE

Skin is the largest organ in the body, and is divided into three layers: epidermis, dermis, and subcutaneous tissue.

The epidermis is the superficial outer layer. When viewed under a microscope, it is stratified into four distinct layers. The top layer is called the stratum corneum, or horny layer, which is very thin but supple and resilient. This layer prevents the entrance of microorganisms and toxic substances. The bottom or basal layer of the epidermis is where actively dividing cells form new cells that migrate upward to replace cells that have sloughed off the horny layer. By the time they reach the surface, these cells are dead. They form a substance called *keratinized protein*, which needs water to look and feel smooth, moist and supple. This dead top layer is constantly sloughing off and replacing itself with young cells from the lower layers, but as the skin ages, young cell production slows down. When this new skin surfaces, the cells are much thicker and more tightly packed. They retain much less moisture than they did when you were younger, giving skin a dull, dry appearance.

The dermis contains the sweat and oil glands, hair follicles, blood vessels, fat glands, and nerve endings in a strong, supportive structure of connective protein fibers called collagen and elastin. Collagen gives skin the ability to stretch, and elastin enables it to spring back into shape. Your skin becomes less resilient and begins to sag, and fine lines and wrinkles begin to appear when this network of collagen and elastin breaks down. As we age, oil and sweat-producing glands begin to slow down their production.

THE PINCH TEST

Place your hand flat on a table, palm facing down. Using the thumb and forefinger, pinch a fold of loose skin on the back of your hand for a few seconds, then let go. Note the time it takes the pinched area to return to normal; this gives you an idea of your skin's relative age. See times listed below.

- Men and women age 10 to 29: 0 seconds
- 30-39: women 1 second; men less than ½ second
- 40-49: women 3 seconds; men 1 second
- 50-59: women 12 seconds; men 4 seconds
- 60-69: women 21 seconds; men 20 seconds
- Over 70: women 1 minute; men 43 seconds

The subcutaneous tissue, located below the dermis, contains fat cells, which store energy and helps conserve body heat. Blood vessels form a network of arteries and veins throughout the subcutaneous tissue and into the dermis.

But don't despair; you *can* keep your skin looking at least 10 years younger than it really is chronologically. Even if your skin is less than perfect, arming yourself with the following awareness will help you win the war on wrinkles, avoiding, improving or eliminating virtually *all* signs of aging on the skin.

AGING TIMETABLE OF NEGLECTED SKIN

Age 25-30: The skin begins to lose moisture; the first tell-tale signs of laugh lines appear.

Age 30-35: Crow's feet begin to appear; laugh lines become more pronounced; undereye area becomes baggy and puffy.

Age 35-40: Oil production slows down and skin becomes dry and papery looking; the jaw line begins to blur.

Age 40-50: Face begins to sag and drop; double chin and jowls develop; the neck becomes crepey; skin color becomes uneven; expression lines turn into full-fledged wrinkles.

Age 50+: New wrinkles develop; the face continues to sag and fall; skin looks mummified.

Three Main Reasons Skin Looks Older Than It Has To

It may seem like the skin experts talk about dozens of different reasons why skin sags and bags, developing lines and wrinkles, but they all boil down to one of three factors: 1. Heredity; 2. Environment; 3. Bad Habits.

— HEREDITY —

Unless you were very careful to select your parents for good-skin genes, this is the single, most important factor in wrinkling. It is also the only one you can't control. Your ancestry plays a large part in how your skin ages. Fair-haired people of Nordic or Celtic descent usually will have lighter, thinner skin, which produces less oil, burns more easily and wrinkles earlier than darker skin. The darker and thicker the skin is, the stronger it is. Blacks, Asians and Caucasians of Mediterranean descent have dark skin that looks younger longer because it has more pigment, which protects collagen from skin-damaging ultraviolet rays. Dark skin is also oilier, so it doesn't dry out as easily or wrinkle as quickly as lighter skin.

Because America's ethnic background is so diverse, most of our ancestors originally came from many different parts of the world, so it may be harder to determine exactly how your skin will react based on heredity. You can, however, look at your parents and both sets of grandparents to get an idea of what's in store for you.

— ENVIRONMENT—

Many environmental aspects, such as climate, humidity, and temperature, adversely affect your skin. But the most damaging force affecting the skin, causing its premature aging and increasing the risk for skin cancer, is ultraviolet radiation. Exposure to the sun's ultraviolet rays is the number one cause of aging skin. Many doctors believe that biological age has nothing to do with aging skin—they say that if we were never exposed to sunlight, our skin would be as smooth and youthful looking at 50 as it was as a teenager. Compare the skin underneath your upper arm with the skin on the back of your hands or forearms.

While sunlight promotes the healthy synthesis of vitamin D in the skin, as well as having beneficial effects on mental well-being, excessive amounts can produce hazardous consequences. One acute reaction is sunburn. That seemingly "healthy" tan is anything but healthy. There is no such thing as a safe tan—a tan is really a radiation burn. Sunlight reacts with oxygen in the skin cells, creating free radicals—unstable oxygen molecules—which damage cell membranes, the fats and proteins the cells need to function, and the RNA and DNA they need to replicate. This is a chronic sun reaction called photoaging, and it damages your skin even more rapidly than conventional aging. The sun destroys collagen by passing through the epidermis to the dermis, where it attacks the collagen in the dermal tissues. This dries the skin out and causes it to harden. This can lead to a condition called keratosis, which is a precursor of skin cancer.

Other chronic reactions are skin disorders, such as brown patches, red spidery veins, and warty growths, as well as more life-threatening reactions, including skin diseases such as melanomas and other skin cancers. Tyrosine, an amino acid, improves the skin's natural resistance to the damaging effects of the sun.

The damage caused by the sun is cumulative over the years. Serious skin problems faced in mid-life have most likely been caused by overexposure while young. But research shows that regular and consistent use of sunscreens prevents further damage while allowing your skin time to repair itself.

Of course, unless you're a vampire or live like one, it's pretty hard to avoid the sun completely. What can you do? First, avoid prolonged direct exposure to the sun. This means either limiting those long, lazy days spent worshipping the sun or eliminating them altogether and substituting other face-saving activities. If the word "vacation" means a trip to the beach, at least spend your time moving around. Don't just sit there. Your blood will circulate faster, supplying nutrients to your skin's cells more efficiently, and you'll minimize exposure to sand-reflected sun rays. When you are going to be exposed to the sun, wear adequate clothing, a hat that shades your face, and sunglasses to help protect the thinner, delicate skin around your eyes.

If you are going to be exposed to direct sunlight for more than a few minutes, wear a sunscreen with an SPF of 15 or higher. Most sunscreens uses PABA, which stops ultraviolet B (UVB) rays, which are the type that cause sunburn. But PABA-sunscreens won't stop ultraviolet A (UVA) rays, which penetrate to the deepest layers of the skin and damage collagen. You need to select a sunscreen containing both PABA and oxybenzone. The newest sunscreen formulations also contain antioxidants—vitamins C and E—which help counter damage from the free radicals produced by sun damage. Be aware that the sun protection factor listed on the bottle (such as SPF 15) refers only to the UVB protection. Their protection against UVA rays is the equivalent of a 2. This means that even though you won't burn as quickly, your skin is still getting radiation damage from UVA rays. Even if you are only going to be minimally exposed to the sun, such as when driving any distance in your car, wear your sunscreen. UVA rays can penetrate glass, so even though you're in the car, you're still catching some rays. Also, remember that the winter sun reflecting off snow can be just as harmful as the summer sun, so wear your sunscreen and sunblock when skiing or participating in other outdoor winter sports.

While it's not practical to wear a sunblock over your entire body, sunblocks do just what the name implies—block out the sun. Use a sunblock containing zinc oxide or titanium dioxide. Some sunblocks are available in many fun colors, so you can choose one to coordinate with or complement your beachwear or outdoor apparel.

Take two aspirin with lots of cold water **before** your skin starts resembling a lobster. Continue taking aspirin every four hours during your exposure to the sun. Besides its pain-relieving property, aspirin helps prevent ultraviolet damage by slowing down prostaglandin production, a hormonelike fatty acid that is part of the skin's inflammation-producing mechanism. Some experts believe that taking aspirin may help promote a better tan, as well.

ALBEDO

Albedo is the measure of light reflected from various surfaces. Remember that black surfaces absorb the sun's rays while light surfaces reflect them. This light-reflective quality of white surfaces is why you'll burn on a sugar-sand beach even when you're under an umbrella; you're still receiving up to 50 percent of the sun's burning rays. Familiarize yourself with these common albedoes: Snow reflects 90 percent; water 50 percent; sand 40 percent; concrete 40 percent; grass 25 percent.

If you have managed to acquire a sunburn despite all your precautions, use cold compresses to relieve the pain and dissipate body heat. Take a cool bath and apply cold milk compresses to the burned areas; the lactic acid in the milk has healing properties. If you prefer, you may soak a washcloth in a bowl of ice cubes filled with equal parts of milk and water, then apply gently to the sunburned areas.

If you simply must have that golden tan, try using a self-tanning product. It is important to exfoliate the skin before application of these products because dead skin cells will grab color quickly, resulting in blotchy, uneven color. After exfoliating, apply the product evenly over the body and wait while color develops. Be careful while spreading it over elbows, knees and around the feet, as the skin there is much thicker and absorbs color more quickly. After applying, carefully wash the palms of your hands—tanned palms look very strange. Better yet, wear gloves during application, then use a cotton pad to apply the product to the backs of your hands.

New Uses For An Old Standby

Recent studies show that old standby, petroleum jelly, to be more than merely an effective barrier against moisture evaporation. When damaged skin was coated with a layer of the jelly, rather than merely sitting on the surface, the petrolatum actually became incorporated into the cellular lipids, aiding in repair.

Other studies show that repeated applications of petroleum jelly helped to increase the skin's thickness as well as providing extra protection against the sun's damaging ultraviolet rays.

Your heredity also plays a part in how your skin reacts to sunlight exposure. Remember that dark skin has more pigment to protect the collagen from damaging sunlight. A blue-eyed blonde or redhead will burn eight times faster than a black woman. Australia's pioneers came mostly from Celtic stock, so it is not surprising that Australia has the world's highest rate of skin cancer. Other areas with high skin cancer rates are the Sunbelt States—Florida, Texas, Hawaii, and the Southwestern states. Because of their balmy climates, people tend to spend even more time out of doors, thus escalating their sun exposure.

The craggy, weather-beaten look may have been attractive on Gary Cooper and John Wayne in those old westerns, but it definitely will not look pretty on you. If you have spent a great deal of time in the sun since you were young, you may have more than just leathery skin and wrinkles to worry about. You may have developed uneven brown patches on face, chest, arms and hands. These hyperpigmented areas are known as liver spots, but they have nothing to do with age. Unfortunately, there is nothing you can do to keep them from appearing, but they can be removed by cryosurgery (a freezing process), electrosurgery (using a needle propelled by electricity), or chemosurgery (a chemical peel). These processes must be performed by a licensed professional or dermatologist.

Other environmental factors that affect your skin are humidity, temperature, wind, and pollution.

Humidity and Temperature

Heating and air conditioning greatly affect the skin's moisture content. Your skin's softness is directly related to its water content. Heat draws moisture from the skin and causes evaporation of surface oils and sweat. Air conditioning reduces humidity in the air and causes the skin to lose moisture. The end result in both cases is skin dehydration. The acid mantle protecting your skin isn't as oily as when you were younger (remember that oil production slows down as you age), so it is not as effective a barrier against moisture evaporation.

The solution? Use a humidifier at home during summer and winter months when heating and air conditioning are necessary. If you don't have a humidifier, place large pans of water on top of your heater or air conditioner. Humidity levels in the air rise as the water evaporates. You'll know when there's enough moisture in the air you're breathing because your throat won't feel dry on awakening.

LOVELY HANDS

Hands not only help you express yourself, they say a lot about you as well. Scruffy, ill-tended hands can destroy the youthful image you have worked so hard to attain. Use a gentle, superfatted soap and rinse thoroughly. Gently pat your hands dry, then use a hand cream. Keep a bottle of hand lotion on your desk; paper handling can strip oils from your hands as quickly as cold weather.

If you don't like creaming your hands after washing them, give your hands a beauty treatment at night. Buy a pair of white cotton gloves. Before turning off the bedside light, stroke petroleum jelly all over your hands, concentrating on any dry, scaly areas, then pull the gloves on. While you sleep, the jelly will soothe and rejuvenate the skin. Apply sunscreen to the backs of your hands before going out—remember that your hands are as exposed to the elements as your face.

Don't neglect your nails. A common misconception is that nails are composed of dead cells. Nails are a living part of the body and should be moisturized and conditioned just like the rest of your skin in order to stay healthy and strong.

Green plants are a great way to add moisture to the air, besides being soothing and pleasant to look at. While you're spritzing their leaves, don't forget to spritz yourself with mineral water. This works like a humidifier, plumping the skin and making fine lines and wrinkles less noticeable.

Spritzing your face is also a great way to add moisture to dry environments when you can't avoid prolonged exposure to heating or cooling systems, such as at the office, in public places, or while flying.

The cabin compression and air conditioning environment in an airplane is very unfriendly to your skin. If you're a frequent flier, you can turn your flight time into a face-saving mini-vacation by using these travel tips: Apply a moisturizer before embarking. Take a small travel container with your favorite eye oil and gently pat it around your eyes between takeoff and landing. Carry your spritzer with you and use it frequently. Instead of indulging in an in-flight cocktail, ask for a mineral water instead. If it's a long trip, drink lots and lots of mineral water.

Wind

If you've ever had a windburn, you know it can hurt as much as a sunburn. Too much exposure to wind can make your skin feel dry as well as robbing it of precious moisture. To minimize wind damage, wear a skin cream containing lanolin in addition to your regular moisturizer. This will help seal your skin from the drying effects of the wind.

Pollution

You may have dealt successfully with all the other environmental influences in your surroundings, but if you live in a big city with poor air quality, you must also take precautions against pollution. You may not be able to see pollution, but it can eat away at your skin. Combat it by sloughing your skin on a weekly basis. If you can afford it, have a professional facial weekly.

— BAD HABITS —

There's an indefinable something about being slightly naughty that appeals to all of us. Certain bad habits seem to add a rakish, devil-may-care spice to life. But for the sake of your skin (and health), there are some bad habits you are just going to have to eliminate from your life. Among them, the most skin and health damaging are cigarette smoking and alcohol abuse. We've already discussed the hazards of sunbathing, so we won't cover that again. Other bad habits (some may surprise you) are abusive weight-loss diets, poor skin care habits, and facial expressions. Not only are these bad habits not particularly glamorous, they constitute facial abuse, so stop them now.

Cigarette Smoking

There is a plethora of information about the health risks of smoking, so we won't cover that here. What we will tell you is that smoking is one of the skin's worst enemies. Smokers' skin ages almost twice as fast as the skin of nonsmokers after the age of 30. Smoking impairs blood circulation, depriving skin of oxygen-rich blood and nutrients, causing lack of color and a pasty, sallow-looking skin. It also causes severe dehydration and severely depletes vitamins A, C and B complex, as well as such minerals as potassium, zinc, and calcium.

Smokers develop early wrinkles, crepey skin, and dark circles and bags under the eyes. Constantly pursing their lips to suck in smoke encourages lip lines, and smokers develop deeper, earlier crow's-feet than nonsmokers because they're constantly squinting to protect their eyes from cigarette smoke. The film stars of the '30s and '40s may have seemed glamorous smoking on the movie screens, but the reality—squinting, watering eyes; muddy, sallow, parched skin; cigarette dangling from wrinkled lips—how glamorous does that sound? To get and keep a fresh, glowing complexion, stop now.

Yeast's Rising Role in Anti-Aging

A live yeast cell derivative called skin respiratory factor (SRF), the active ingredient in the over-the-counter hemorrhoid shrinker, Preparation H, encourages tissue healing by increasing cell oxygenation. This increases production of collagen and elastin in the skin, which in turn, minimizes fine lines and wrinkles. The increased oxygenation also improves skin texture and tone.

Preparation H also contains shark liver oil. Like other fish liver oils, shark liver oil contains lots of Vitamin A, whose by-product is the famous wrinkle-reducer, Retin-A. For years, some of the world's most glamorous models have included Preparation H in their top-secret, anti-aging weapon arsenal. You don't have to rush out and buy a tube of Preparation H, though—there are increasingly available products on the market that contain SRF.

Another yeast extract, beta glucan, also stimulates the skin's production of collagen. It, too, is available in certain lines of skin-care products. Always be sure to read the product label before purchasing.

Alcohol Abuse

Excessive alcohol intake, like cigarette smoking and prolonged sun exposure, ages the skin rapidly. Alcohol impairs vitamin metabolism, robbing the skin of the same nutrients that cigarette smoking does. It also derails a normal appetite, causing heavy drinkers to either eat less or eat the wrong types of food, further depleting their nutritional reserves.

CAFFEINE FIENDS

Your morning wake-up beverage may be robbing you of vital nutrients, causing energy levels to drop and impeding cell production. Like nicotine, caffeine causes severe dehydration of the skin. It depletes vitamins and robs the cells of skin-beautifying oxygen. Switch to a non-caffeinated morning drink. An ideal beverage is orange juice, which contains vitamin C, a collagen-booster, and natural sugars, which will wake you up as effectively as caffeine.

Don't think you can switch to tea, unless it's herbal tea. Though regular black tea contains only half as much caffeine as coffee, it also contains tannin, a substance that impedes the body's absorption of iron.

Other caffeine-containing drinks frequently imbibed include colas, hot chocolate, and other soft drinks. Even some over-the-counter pain-relievers and antihistamines contain anywhere from 75 to 200 milligrams per dose. That's the equivalent of a 6-ounce cup of java.

Like cigarettes, alcohol dehydrates your skin by decreasing the water concentration in the blood. Your body reacts by pulling water from the skin cells into the blood. After a while, this loss of valuable moisture leads to wrinkling.

Heavy drinking damages internal organs, such as the liver, which is responsible for breaking down toxic substances in your body. When the liver becomes toxic, the results show up on the skin, which looks sallow and dull.

Overconsumption of alcohol dilates the blood vessels of the face, leading to spidery, broken blood vessels on the cheeks and nose. This is called the "blush effect." W.C. Fields was certainly a very funny man, but how attractive was that big red nose of his? Only abusive alcohol consumption causes problems. A glass of wine with dinner or an occasional cocktail is fine.

Abusive Dieting

The yo-yo dieting syndrome, crash diets and severely restrictive fad diets can produce nutrient deprivation, greatly harming your skin as well as your body and metabolism.

Prolonged fasting can dehydrate the skin, making it look flaky and sallow. Diet pills and diuretics pull vital water from the cells, including the skin cells. And constant weight gain followed by rapid weight loss doesn't allow the skin time to catch up. It is constantly stretching and shrinking, stretching and shrinking to accommodate these fluctuations in weight. Eventually, the collagen and elastin that form the underlying support for the skin begin to break down. The result is loose, sagging skin. Remember to save your face while dieting and don't try to lose weight too fast.

The experts' recommendation for safe weight loss of two pounds per week is not only good diet sense, it can save your skin as well. While you're safely losing those weekly two pounds, be sure to follow a sensible diet. For a balanced diet, eat fresh vegetables and fruits, high-fiber whole grains, fish, poultry, and complex carbohydrates. Round out this face-loving diet with appropriate vitamin and mineral supplements.

Don't forget to exercise regularly. It increases circulation, oxygenates the blood, and flushes toxins from the body—all good for your skin. See the boxed copy on page 33 for more benefits of exercise. If you have led a very sedentary lifestyle, be sure to consult your physician before embarking on any exercise program.

Poor Skin Care Habits

Poor skin care leads to skin that looks old before its time. Follow the 6-step skin care regimen beginning on page 34.

Facial Expressions

A mobile, expressive face is attractive but certain expressions, when repeated over long periods of time, can cause wrinkles. It is said that these wrinkles add character to the face, but while smile lines around the mouth and laughter crinkles around the eyes show that we are living, feeling creatures who enjoy life, what do those frown lines say about us? Any character such ill-humored lines may add to your face certainly won't enhance your good looks. It takes fewer muscles to smile than to frown, which proves that being grumpy is hard work. Take some laugh breaks throughout the day and learn to smile more, frown less.

HOW EXERCISE BENEFITS YOUR SKIN

- Increases blood circulation, delivering vital nutrients and oxygen to skin cells.

- Helps to increase the production of new cells in the basal layer of the skin. Also speeds up collagen and elastin production.

- Raises skin temperature, which also increases production of collagen.

- Increases the skin's oil- and sweat-gland production, thus slowing down the aging process.

- Eliminates toxins in the body that can dull your skin and cause pimples and other blemishes.

- Encourages perspiration, which helps to flush out toxins, dirt and other impurities from the skin.

- Helps relieve stress, and plays a large part in helping eliminate bad habits such as smoking and excessive drinking, which age the skin rapidly.

- Burns calories, helping you attain and maintain your desired weight goal and avoid drastic weight gain and weight loss, which is very bad for the skin.

Age-Defying, Wrinkle-Reducing Care For Mature Skin

Correct and appropriate skin care can erase five to ten years from your face in just two weeks. Why do we say you'll start seeing dramatic results in only two weeks? Because it takes two weeks for the cells in the horny layer of the epidermis to turn over and be replaced by fresh young cells rising from the basal layer. Religious adherence to the skin-care regimen outlined below will stimulate your basal layer to produce lots of moist new cells.

By correct skin care, we mean scrupulously following the six steps outlined below; they are crucial to achieving a younger-looking complexion. By appropriate skin care, we mean knowing your skin type and using products specifically formulated for it, then modifying the 6-step regimen accordingly. Most people know their skin type. If you are unsure what type your skin is, refer to the box on the next page.

6-STEP REGIMEN FOR — YOUNGER-LOOKING SKIN—

1. *Complete Makeup Removal*
2. *Thorough Cleansing*
3. *Regular Sloughing*
4. *Toning*
5. *Moisturizing and Nourishing*
6. *Stimulating and Firming*

BRIEF OVERVIEW OF SKIN TYPES

OILY SKIN

- Thicker and oilier than dry or combination skin
- Attracts dirt more quickly
- Oily sheen reappears quickly after cleansing
- Coarse texture and large pores
- Sites of teenage skin eruptions may flare up under stress
- Absorbs makeup quickly and causes change in coverage and color
- Stays younger-looking longer

DRY SKIN

- Thin skin with small, fine-grained pores
- Flakes easily as it ages
- Loses elasticity at early age
- Lines and wrinkles appear at early age
- Feels tight and dry after cleansing
- Wrinkles earlier than other skin types

COMBINATION SKIN

- Cheeks are dry with small, fine-grained pores
- T-zone (forehead, nose and chin) is oily with large pores
- Occasional blackheads and blemishes in the T-zone

1. Complete Makeup Removal

The first step in your skin-care regimen is extremely important. **Never, never, never** go to bed with stale makeup, no matter how exhausted you may be. This is especially important if you wear more than just powder or lipstick. Foundation, blusher, and eye makeup must be thoroughly removed before you can follow any of the other steps. Proper makeup removal takes just a minute and makes step two easier.

Makeup on dry or normal skin should be removed with a product specially formulated for your skin type. Stroke it gently all over the face and leave on one minute to loosen makeup, then remove with a washcloth dipped in warm, not hot, water. (Water that is too hot can cause the tiny capillaries in the face to rupture, leaving spidery little red lines around the nose and on the cheeks.) Be very gentle when removing makeup; never pull or tug at your skin. If there are still stubborn remnants of makeup on your face, repeat the process. If your skin tends to be oily or is prone to breakouts, try using a liquid soap replacement.

All skin types should use a specially formulated eye-makeup remover on the gentle tissues of the eye area. Gently stroke on with a cotton ball. Use the reverse side to remove any excess or use a warm, wet washcloth. **Never** use facial tissues to remove eye makeup, as facial tissues are made from wood pulp and are too abrasive for this delicate area. **Never** pull or tug the skin around your eyes. See the section on handling the delicate skin around the eye on page 44.

2. Thorough Cleansing

Now that you have removed all traces of makeup from your face, you are ready to continue with the cleansing process. Makeup removal alone is not enough to clean the skin. Proper cleansing removes accumulated dirt, pollut-ants, and other debris from your skin.

Soap may have done an adequate job of cleansing your face when you were younger, but its alkalinity can make mature skin feel tight and dry. If you feel you absolutely must use soap, choose a super-fatted soap and be sure to rinse your skin several times. Or you may choose to use a liquid soap replacement cleanser specially formulated for normal to dry skin or a cream-type cleanser for very dry skins. Oily skins may choose to use a soap with cleansing grains or pumice.

Wet your face and apply the cleanser, working it gently over the face. Rinse thoroughly in tepid water. Never use very hot or very cold water to rinse your face; broken capillaries can result. If your next step is sloughing, you don't need to dry your face. If your next step is toning, gently pat face semi-dry.

3. Sloughing

Now that your face is immaculately clean and glowing, you're ready for the next step. Every skin needs to be sloughed on a regular basis, especially when it begins to age. **Why?** As we discussed earlier in the book, production of new cells in maturing skin slows way down. When the cells do reach the outer layer of the epidermis, they are much thicker and more tightly packed. As they accumulate on the surface of your skin, they block new cells from surfacing. They also accumulate cellular debris and waste. The longer these old, dead cells lie there, the duller and drier your complexion will become. Exfoliation removes this cellular debris and stimulates the growth of new cells.

When: Unless you use a very gentle exfoliant, daily sloughing may be too much. Try exfoliating three or four times a week. If this leaves your skin feeling raw, decrease to once or twice weekly. If your skin is extremely sensitive, decrease to once every 10 days or every two weeks. You don't want to flay the skin right off your face. If you have combination skin, slough the drier cheek area once or twice weekly, and the T-zone three or four times a week or daily, if desired. Men only need to slough their forehead and nose; they exfoliate the rest of their face every time they shave.

VITAMIN UPDATE

As you age, a phenomenon called "cross-linking" occurs. The strings of collagen protein become tangled from years of accumulated damage by exposure to sun, tobacco smoke, chemicals, and other toxins. The end result: skin loses elasticity, becoming stiff and rigid. The solution: antioxidant vitamins C, A and E. They help prevent or minimize cross-linking damage at the cellular level. Another anti-oxidant, Beta-carotene, a precursor of vitamin A, has been shown to prevent or slow development of skin cancer.

How: First, wet your face. Work your fingertips into the exfoliant, then move them gently over your face. Start at the nose and work out to the cheeks, then up the cheeks to the temples. Always use upward strokes during any cleansing, toning or exfoliating action. Do the chin, neck and forehead last. You may also use a mildly abrasive store-bought cleanser formulated for your skin type, or make your own exfoliant, as in the following recipe.

Skin-Loving Enzyme Peel

Put a tablespoon of fresh papaya (or fresh pineapple) into a blender. Add a teaspoon of honey, a half-teaspoon sunflower or sesame seeds, and a few crushed almonds, then blend. The effective ingredient in papaya is an enzyme called papain, which actually helps to dissolve damaged collagen and encourages the body to produce healthy new collagen fibers. Bromelain, found in fresh pineapple, is another enzyme that has the same effect on the skin's collagen as papain. If you want to cut down preparation time, you can still get great benefits from these skin-loving enzymes by simply rubbing the skin with a slice or two of fresh pineapple or mashed papaya for one minute, then rinsing thoroughly.

When you are done exfoliating, rinse your skin thoroughly with warm water. Gently pat skin with a soft towel. **Never** rub, tug or pull the skin; this will stretch and weaken the collagen and elastin in your skin. Don't completely dry the skin; leave it slightly damp and proceed to the next step.

4. Toning

Using the proper toner will smooth your skin and tighten the pores, causing fine lines and wrinkles to be less noticeable. Toner accomplishes this by slightly irritating the skin, which is the tingle you feel when applying it. Skin surrounding the pores swells and blocks the pore opening from view, making fine lines and wrinkles less apparent.

Oily skin can use an astringent, which has some alcohol content and is more drying than a toner. Normal to dry skin should use a skin toner without alcohol. Saturate a cotton ball or pad and gently sweep across the face, using upward strokes. Your skin is now prepared to receive a moisturizer if you're performing this step in the morning, or a nourishing cream at night.

5. Moisturizing and Nourishing

First, you should know what a moisturizer can and cannot do. Despite the name, they do not make your skin moist. What they do is trap water on your skin. This is why you don't want to dry your face completely before applying moisturizer. Some moisturizers act as humectants by attracting moisture from the environment to your skin. Moisturizer's main function is to seal water into your skin and prevent it from evaporating into the air. The moistened skin plumps out, minimizing small lines and wrinkles. A secondary function is to replace some of the oils lost during the cleansing, sloughing and toning steps.

A physiologically active moisturizer penetrates the epidermis to moisturize the cells below, increasing cell turnover, improving skin texture and diminishing tiny lines and wrinkles. But don't expect miracles—deep grooves and heavily etched wrinkles will not be affected. No over-the-counter skin-care product will erase wrinkles, despite advertising claims. But when used consistently, they will improve the surface appearance of your skin by plumping the surface skin cells, filling in lines and giving your skin a healthy glow.

"Dryness of the skin is primarily due to loss of water from the skin's horny outer layer and insufficient movement of moisture upward from lower tissue layers. In experiments with thin sections of dry and brittle horny tissue, contact with various 'fatty' materials such as lanolin or vegetable oil did not restore the pliability of the material even when contact was prolonged. On the other hand, immersing the tissue in water or maintaining it in humid air did."

—AMA Book of Skin and Hair Care

For more dramatic results than you can get with non-prescription products, consult your dermatologist for information about Retin-A and what it can do for you. Understand that "Retin-A" is a trade name; the product is also known as retinoic acid, vitamin A acid, or tretinoin. Preparations containing similar-sounding ingredients, like "retinyl" or such spellings, are merely attempts to make you think you're going to get the same effects as with Retin-A. Don't be fooled. At time of publication of this book, Retin-A is still **only** available by prescription, and because of its potency (retinoids as a class are teratogenic and can cause birth defects), it is unlikely the FDA will release it for over-the-counter sales.

But don't despair—alpha-hydroxy acids, such as lactic acid and glycolic acid, are available without prescription and are almost as effective as Retin-A, without the side effects. Again, there is a problem with the many cosmetic companies that have jumped on the bandwagon, offering preparations containing as little as two or three percent alpha-hydroxy acids. In concentrations as low as these, the products are virtually ineffective. Look for concentrations of at least five percent, and preferably higher. The higher the concentration, however, the greater the chance sensitive skin will feel irritated by the stinging effect. If the higher concentrations are too irritating for your skin, start with one of the lower concentrations and gradually work up to the higher levels.

To moisturize your skin (daytime): Wet your skin, then gently blot off excess, leaving skin damp. Place a dot of moisturizer the size of a dime in your palm, then dot on your face. Gently spread the moisturizer across the skin.

To nourish your skin (before bed): Dot an emollient-rich night cream over your face and smooth in. The extra-rich ingredients in a nourishing cream would be too heavy to use during the daytime; they work best at night while your body is repairing itself during sleep.

VITAMIN C CREAM

Vitamin C strengthens and rejuvenates collagen. A topical application of cream containing vitamin C can help your skin to synthesize new collagen.

All skin types need to use moisturizer, even oily skin types. Moisture has nothing to do with oil. The surface moisture in your skin is composed of water from the sweat glands and oil from the sebaceous glands. As the skin ages, the sebum and oil producing glands slow down, which means that not enough of the skin's own natural moisturizers reach the surface to protect the skin. The skin's own ability to retain moisture lessens with each year. Because oily skin has more of a protective barrier against moisture loss than dry skin, it ages more slowly than dry skin. But we're talking about replacing moisture in the skin, not oil, so even if your skin is oily, you must still moisturize. There are moisturizers available that are specially formulated for oily skins, so you have no excuse to skip this step.

6. Stimulating and Firming

Masks stimulate and firm your skin through several actions: They temporarily tighten the skin by slightly irritating it, thus minimizing enlarged pores. Masks draw out and remove dead, flaky cellular debris and other impurities, making skin look smoother, clearer and fresher. They help heal minor blemishes and make wrinkles seem to disappear, at least temporarily. All skin types will benefit by regular use of this step. Normal-to-dry and combination skins may use a gel-type mask, which helps lock in moisture. Oily skins befit by using a clay or mud-type mask. Also, clay masks are particularly beneficial for older skins because the clay is rich in natural minerals that draw impurities from the skin, which can lead to blemishes, blackheads and whiteheads. The clay pulls out cellular debris while tightening the pores and stimulating circulation. Because clay can have a drying effect, choose the kind of clay that's best for your skin type. Oily and combination skins should use green, dark brown or mudlike clay. Dry or sensitive skin should use white clay, which is very gentle. All skin types can use rose clay.

When applying the mask, be careful to avoid the delicate skin tissue around the eye area. Be sure to include the skin on your throat when masking; it will tighten and tone this area. Use masks once a week; more often during summer months.

Make your own mask: Dissolve one package of unflavored gelatin in 1/2 cup of boiling water. Mash four or five strawberries and add to gelatin. Chill until mixture begins to thicken—approximately one hour. Apply to face for ten minutes, then rinse with cool water.

EXTREMELY DRY SKIN

Many experts think that extremely dry skin may be caused by a low-grade skin inflammation. Hydrocortisone creams, available without prescription, can penetrate the epidermis, hydrate cells, and reduce the inflammation. Check with your dermatologist to see if you have this skin condition.

SPECIAL CARE FOR THE —DELICATE EYE AREA—

This delicate area requires special handling and treatment. The skin of the eye zone is the thinnest on your body and has almost no fatty, plumping padding. It is more prone to developing fine lines and wrinkles because it lacks the sweat and oil glands that produce the skin's natural defense barrier. This delicate tissue is also prone to sagging and bagging because of the muscle surrounding the eye, which is circular and has no cross support. Rubbing your eyes, pulling the eyelid to apply eye makeup, and any other pulling or tugging movement weakens the muscle surrounding the eye and causes sagging of the entire eye area. Constant squinting encourages fine lines around the eye and between the brows, so be sure to wear sunglasses outdoors and stay away from eye irritants, such as cigarette smoke, soot and dust.

THE EYES HAVE IT

Raw potato slices make soothing compresses to reduce swelling and puffiness around the eyes. Put the slices between two flat pieces of cotton and place on the lids for about 10 minutes. Other puffy eye relievers include milk-soaked cotton pads placed on the eyes for a few minutes. Or use witch hazel on cotton pads to refresh eyes and reduce swelling. Of course, the familiar old standby—tea bags, either regular or chamomile—are effective, too. Steep the bags for a few minutes in boiling water. Squeeze out excess water and smooth bags flat before placing on the eyes for 10 to 15 minutes. Cucumber slices (hold the salad dressing) make wonderfully soothing eye compresses.

To avoid weakening the skin around the eyes, use your middle, ring or pinkie finger when applying any creams, oils or makeup to the eye area. Your index (pointer) finger is too strong and can stretch the delicate skin around the eye area.

The best way to remove eye makeup: Always begin with the finger at the outer corner and move inward toward nose. Continue the circle around over the eyelid and back to the outer edge.

The same procedure should be used when applying eye creams. Do not to get the cream too close to the lash area—it can cause puffiness and irritation. Instead, gently pat the cream along the edge of the bone surrounding the eye socket. As the cream penetrates the skin, it will seep upward, moisturizing the area beneath the lashes. Don't neglect to lubricate the upper lid.

Do not use your face moisturizer on the delicate eye area. It may contain certain fragrances, emollients and emulsifiers that can be potentially irritating to the eyes. Choose an eye cream formulated without these ingredients. Be sure to use your eye cream or oil twice daily after cleansing.

VITAMIN E CREAM

Application of a 5 percent vitamin E cream can result in a more than 50 percent reduction in the length and depth of crow's-feet. Look for moisturizers that have vitamin E (tocopherol) near the top of the ingredients list. Or make your own by adding the oil from a vitamin E capsule to a small amount of eye cream and mixing well. Don't use the oil from the capsule directly on the skin as it can cause some irritation.

—OTHER SKIN PROBLEMS—

The Throat Area

While you are rejuvenating the skin on your face, don't neglect your throat. Crepey skin on your neck can destroy the youthful look your face projects. Like your eyes, the skin on your throat needs special care. It contains no oil glands and, like the eye area, you must use a cream specially formulated for the neck and throat area. These creams contain special tightening agents as well as moisturizers. Apply with long, sweeping motions, starting at the collarbone and continuing toward the chin line.

Blackheads

Unfortunately, this is one skin problem that does not necessarily go away with age. To help dry up oily blackheads and speed their departure, swab the affected area with milk of magnesia and leave on overnight. Squeezing a blackhead is not recommended; you can do permanent damage to the surrounding skin tissue. But, if you simply cannot wait for it to go away of its own accord, follow these instructions for safer removal: Soften the skin around the blackhead with a washcloth that has been dipped in warm to hot water, then wrung out. Hold the washcloth on the blackhead for a few seconds, then repeat the procedure twice more. Now, hold a tissue in each hand and gently exert pressure with both forefingers on either side of the blackhead, being very careful not to pinch the skin, or scarring could result. Now the plug, having been loosened by the warmth of the hot washcloth, should be easy to remove. After you have removed it, be sure to pat an astringent or witch hazel over the pore to cleanse it and to encourage it to close. The section on natural skin preparations contains some recipes that will assist you in the blackhead removal process.

Baggy or Hooded Eyes

Those mail pouches you may be carrying around under your eyes could be hereditary, the result of yo-yo dieting, or an immoderate lifestyle that includes too much alcohol or too little sleep. Unlike puffiness under the eyes, bags don't go away after you've been awake for a while. These pouches are actually pockets of fat pads that bulge through the delicate skin around the eye. If they are hereditary and not something that an improved lifestyle can change, the solution is a surgical process called blepharoplasty, which can be performed separately or as part of a face-lift.

Hooded eyes can make you look years older than you are. The hoods are caused when the eyebrows begin to fall forward, pushing the skin of the eyelid forward as well. You may elect to have a plastic surgeon correct the problem. Artfully applied makeup and reshaping the eyebrows can also help conceal or modify the problem. The makeup section contains additional tips on how to use makeup to achieve eye-opening results.

Dark Circles Under the Eyes

Dark circles are caused by blood passing through veins close to the skin's surface. As you get older and the skin under yours eyes becomes thinner and more transparent, the circles get darker.

To counteract this problem, look for eye creams that contain a hint of color to camouflage dark circles while smoothing fine lines. The makeup section a little later in the book contains some helpful tips on how to camouflage dark circles.

NATURAL, EFFECTIVE
— SKIN PREPARATIONS—

Make your own skin care products at home for a fraction of the cost of store-bought preparations. You'll know exactly what went into each skin care preparation and will never have to worry about allergic reactions to synthetic dyes, perfumes, chemical additives, or preservatives. Because they are all-natural and contain no preservatives, make small quantities of each preparation and refrigerate any remaining product, especially those containing perishable foods, such as milk, eggs, wheat germ, etc. Buy only fresh ingredients for use in your skin preparations; never use leftovers, which may oxidize when exposed to air.

The following recipes contain familiar ingredients found in most kitchens. Natural food stores are a good place to buy pesticide-free fruits and vegetables, cold-pressed oils and natural eggs and milk. Other ingredients can be obtained at your local health food store, or check with a pharmacy for such items as hydrous lanolin, tincture of benzoin, and glycerine. Recipes calling for a certain floral or herbal water may require an additional step. Prepare an infusion of the flower or herb, let it cool, then use it in the recipe.

Some recipes have been handed down for generations and have stood the test of time; others are based on the latest knowledge about the ingredients' beautifying properties. Whatever the case, although the following recipes have been tested and perform their intended job beautifully, it may take a while to discover which formulas work best for your particular skin. All measurements given are approximate, since climate can alter textures. You may need to experiment, adjusting measurements, until the formula meets your own special requirements.

Don't let the simplicity of ingredients and preparation fool you—these products are as effective and beneficial as the most expensive store-bought cream containing unpronounceable ingredients.

— CLEANSERS —

Almond Cleansing Cream

4 ounces oil of sweet almonds
1 ounce hydrous lanolin
1 ounce petroleum jelly

Melt the lanolin and petroleum jelly in a double boiler over low heat. When melted, remove from heat and beat in oil of sweet almonds. Cool before using. Massage over face and neck, removing with warm, wet washcloth. Put the remainder in a jar and store in a cool place.

Almond Meal Cleanser

1/2 cup oil of sweet almonds
1/2 cup corn or powdered oatmeal
1/2 cup grated or powdered castile soap

Combine dry ingredients. Stir in oil until completely blended. Mixture will be thick, but do not add any liquid. Store in covered jar in refrigerator. To use, put a spoonful in palm of hand and add just enough water to bring to a creamy consistency. Then apply to the face with upward, sweeping motions. Remove with warm, wet washcloth, and rinse thoroughly.

Apricot Cleansing Cream

4 tablespoons apricot oil
2 tablespoons sesame seed oil
2 tablespoons sweet (unsalted) butter
1 tablespoon distilled water

Combine all ingredients in a bowl and beat until completely smooth and creamy. You may also use a blender. To use, massage the cleanser over your face and neck. Remove with warm water and washcloth. Store in covered jar in refrigerator between uses.

Lemon Cleansing Cream

6 tablespoons vegetable shortening
2 tablespoons freshly squeezed lemon juice

Strain any pulp from the lemon juice, and beat into the vegetable shortening until smooth. Smooth over the skin with fingertips. Gently remove with warm, wet washcloth. This cleanser is good for normal skins. Store remainder in refrigerator between uses.

Olive Cleansing Cream

4 tablespoons olive oil
2 tablespoons sesame seed oil
2 tablespoons vegetable shortening
2 drops essence of elder, chamomile or rose

Combine all ingredients in a bowl and beat until completely smooth and creamy. Excellent for use before a warm bath. Leave on during bath to allow oils to penetrate skin. Remove with warm, wet washcloth and rinse skin thoroughly. Store remaining cream in a covered jar in the refrigerator.

Orange Wake-up Cleanser

6 tablespoons petroleum jelly
1 tablespoon freshly squeezed orange juice
1/4 teaspoon borax

Strain pulp from orange juice and heat over a low flame. Remove from heat and mix in the borax. Meanwhile, in a separate pot, melt the petroleum jelly over low heat. When completely melted, stir in the orange juice-borax mixture until mixture reaches a creamy consistency. Massage over face and neck, then remove with washcloth dipped in warm water. This cleanser is particularly good for oily skin. Refrigerate.

--- SKIN SLOUGHERS ---

Baking Soda Exfoliator

1 teaspoon olive or almond oil
Baking soda

Pour the oil into the palm of your hand and add enough baking soda to make a thin paste. Apply to face with light, sweeping strokes, being careful to avoid the delicate skin around the eyes. Using small circular motions, massage into the skin on forehead, cheeks and chin. Be careful not to massage any area for more than 10 or 15 seconds, particularly if skin is very sensitive. Rinse thoroughly and pat the skin dry. Follow with toner and moisturizer.

Gelatin Exfoliater

1 package unflavored gelatin
3 tablespoons distilled water

Mix the water into the gelatin until it forms a paste. Apply this paste to the skin and let dry. Remove with warm, wet washcloth and apply moisturizer.

Salt-and-Soap Exfoliator

Castile soap
2 tablespoons sea salt

Splash your face with warm water, then work soap into a rich lather. Add one teaspoon salt and rub palms together. Apply to the skin using light, sweeping strokes, then gently massage forehead, cheeks, and chin. Continue massaging the soap-and-salt mixture into the skin for one minute, adding the rest of the salt as necessary. Rinse thoroughly and pat dry. Follow with freshener or toner, unless skin feels too sensitive.

— ASTRINGENTS —

Tingling Mint Astringent
For normal skin

1 pint cider vinegar
1 pint distilled water
1 cup peppermint leaves

In a large pot, bring all ingredients to a boil. Remove from heat, let cool and pour into a glass jar. Steep for five days. Strain mixture and use.

Rose Water Astringent
For normal to dry skin

1/4 teaspoon boric acid powder
1 1/4 teaspoon witch hazel
2 ounces glycerine

2 ounces rubbing alcohol
1 1/2 ounce rose water
1/4 teaspoon benzoin

Dissolve the boric acid in the witch hazel, then add other ingredients. Mix thoroughly and store in cool, dark place. Stroke gently over skin with cotton pad.

Bracing Sage Astringent

For normal skin

1/2 cup dried sage
1/2 cup alcohol
1 teaspoon glycerine
3 tablespoons witch hazel
1/4 teaspoon benzoin
1/4 teaspoon boric acid powder

Steep the sage in the rubbing alcohol for one week, then strain. Dissolve boric acid powder in the witch hazel, then add glycerine and benzoin. Finally, add the sage extract, and store in glass jar.

Australian Tea Tree Astringent

For normal-to-oily or troubled skin

1 ounce spirits of camphor
2 1/2 ounces glycerine
4 ounces rubbing alcohol
2 ounces distilled water
2 teaspoons tea tree oil

Mix all ingredients together, adding the water last. Shake before using. Apply with cotton pads.

Yankee-Style Astringent

For oily skin

1 ounce apple cider vinegar
1 ounce distilled water

Mix together and apply with cotton pad to face and neck. Refrigerate between uses.

--- TONERS ---

Almond Freshener
For normal skin

3 ounces almond extract
2 ounces witch hazel
1/8 teaspoon alum powder

Combine all ingredients in a bottle. Shake thoroughly before using. To use, saturate a cotton pad and stroke over the face. Refrigerate between uses.

Cucumber Toner I
For normal skin

1 peeled cucumber
3 ounces distilled water
1 teaspoon essence of melissa

Coarsely chop cucumber and put into blender with water and essence of melissa. Puree until blended thoroughly. Saturate a cotton pad with the mixture and gently stroke over the skin. Refrigerate any remaining toner.

Cucumber Toner II
For dry skin

1 peeled cucumber
1 teaspoon witch hazel
1 teaspoon rose water
1 egg white

Grate or shred the cucumber finely. Add witch hazel and rose water. Beat the egg white until frothy, then stir into cucumber mixture. Strain before use. Saturate cotton pad with mixture and gently stroke over skin. Refrigerate any remaining toner.

Gentle Skin Toner

For dry skin

1 ounce mineral oil
2 1/2 ounces glycerine
4 ounces milk of magnesia
4 ounces witch hazel

Stir slowly together all the ingredients; keep in a tightly covered glass bottle and shake before use. Saturate cotton pad with toner and stroke gently over face and throat.

Lavender Skin Toner

2 cups lavender flowers
1 ounce powdered orris root
1 pint vinegar

Steep the lavender flowers and orris root in the vinegar for one month. Strain and dilute with an equal amount of distilled water. Keep in refrigerator.

Old-Fashioned Skin Toner

For dry skin

1 cup rose water
1/4 cup glycerine

Mix rose water and glycerine and pour into bottle. To use, shake bottle thoroughly, then saturate cotton pad with toner and stroke over face and neck.

Rose-Vinegar Freshener

4 cups dried red roses
1/2 cup essence of rose
1 pint vinegar

Place all ingredients in a lidded glass jar and steep for three weeks, shaking frequently. Strain before using and dilute with equal parts of distilled water. Stroke gently over face and throat. Store in refrigerator.

— CREAMS & CONDITIONERS —

Almond Night Cream

3 tablespoons almond oil
2 tablespoons hydrous lanolin
2 tablespoons cocoa butter
2 teaspoons rose water
1/2 teaspoon honey

Put almond oil, lanolin and cocoa butter in a double boiler and heat until the ingredients melt together. Remove from heat and stir in the rose water and honey. Allow to cool, then beat until thoroughly blended. Store in glass container in refrigerator.

Almond Lotion

5 tablespoons distilled water
2 tablespoons glycerine
1 tablespoon witch hazel
1/4 teaspoon almond oil

Combine all ingredient in a bottle. Shake before using, then apply to thoroughly cleansed and toned skin with fingertips.

Apricot Cream

2 tablespoons lanolin
1 tablespoon apricot oil
1 teaspoon lemon juice
3 drops tincture of benzoin

Heat lanolin in a double boiler until melted, then stir in apricot oil and lemon juice. Mix until thoroughly blended, then add the benzoin. Beat again. Store in the refrigerator.

Rich Avocado Conditioner

2 whole eggs
2 egg yolks, beaten
2 tablespoons distilled water
2 teaspoons avocado oil
1 teaspoon glycerine
1/2 teaspoon freshly squeezed lemon juice
1/2 teaspoon cider vinegar

Blend together the glycerine and whole eggs, then add the strained lemon juice. Slowly add the avocado oil until the mixture thickens, then stir in the vinegar. Last, blend in the beaten egg yolks and water very slowly, stirring all the while. Store in refrigerator.

Chapped Skin Cream

6 tablespoons sweet almond oil
2 ounces rose water
1/2 ounce white wax
1 teaspoon cod liver oil

Melt the wax and oils in a double boiler over low heat. When completely melted, remove from heat and slowly add rose water a few drops at a time, thoroughly beating after each addition. Use on rough, dry skin, paying special attention to elbows, knees and chapped hands.

Cucumber Cream

1 peeled cucumber
2 ounces oil of sweet almonds
1/2 ounce white wax

Grate or chop the cucumber very finely. Place the white wax in a double boiler and heat until melted, then add the almond oil. Add the cucumber and cover the pot. Simmer for one hour, then remove from heat. Stir thoroughly, then strain. Refrigerate.

Elder Flower Cream

1 cup elder flowers
1 tablespoon lanolin
6 ounces sweet almond oil

Melt lanolin in a double boiler, then add almond oil, blending well. Add elder flowers; simmer gently for 30 minutes. Cool and strain before use. Refrigerate.

Mature Skin Reviver

1/4 cup apricot oil
4 drops chamomile oil
5 drops carrot seed oil
8 drops geranium oil
5 drops lavender oil
1 drops patchouli oil
2 drops sandalwood oil

Blend the oils together thoroughly. Smooth over the skin before bathing; the warmth of the bath will help the oils penetrate the skin, or use after showering.

Leafy Green Cream

1 cup very finely chopped leafy-type lettuce
1/2 cup lanolin
2 drops rose or geranium oil

Put lanolin in a double boiler and heat until melted. Add lettuce and beat until thoroughly blended. Remove from heat and add the essential oil. Strain; store in refrigerator.

Honey Almond Cream

8 ounces hydrous lanolin
1/2 cup oil of sweet almonds
4 ounces natural honey

Heat the honey in a double boiler. When it is warmed, add the lanolin and heat until melted, then stir in the almond oil. Remove from the heat and beat until creamy. Store in refrigerator.

Old-Fashioned Eye Cream

1 teaspoon beeswax
1 teaspoon mineral oil
1/2 teaspoon lanolin

Melt all ingredients in a double boiler over low heat. Remove from heat and beat until cool. Store in jar in a cool place. Gently pat onto the skin around the eyes.

Strawberry Conditioner

1/2 cup fresh or frozen strawberry juice
1 1/4 teaspoon lanolin
1 1/4 teaspoon finely ground oatmeal

Put lanolin in a double boiler and heat until melted. Stir in oatmeal. When mixture is smooth, add juice and beat until creamy. Store in a glass jar in refrigerator.

Ultra-Rich Eye Cream

2 teaspoons petroleum jelly
1 teaspoon almond oil
50,000 IU Vitamin A from capsules
2,500 IU Vitamin D from capsules
1,200 IU Vitamin E from capsules

Blend almond oil and petroleum together in a small container. Prick open the vitamin capsules and squeeze the contents into the almond-petroleum jelly mixture. Blend thoroughly. Store in refrigerator. Smooth around eye areas before retiring at night.

Essential Oil Skin Reviver

1 ounce wheat germ oil
3 drops each of the following:
orange flower; sage; melissa; sweet
marjoram, and lavender oils

Blend the oils together thoroughly and use as needed.

--- MASKS & FACIALS ---

Almond Mask I

1 egg white
1 tablespoon almonds
1/2 teaspoon freshly squeezed lemon juice

Grind the almonds in a blender or coffee grinder until powdery. Beat the egg white until frothy, then mix in the powdered almonds and lemon juice. Apply to skin with fingertips, avoiding the eyes, and leave on 20 minutes. Remove with warm water and follow with a cool water rinse.

Almond Mask II

4 ounces blanched almonds
1 egg white
1 or 2 tablespoons rose water

Grind the almonds in a blender or coffee grinder until powdery, then add the egg white, unbeaten, and enough rose water to make a paste. Apply to the skin and leave on for 10 minutes. Remove with a warm, wet washcloth.

Avocado Mask

Place half of a ripe avocado in a blender and blend until smooth. Put the avocado in a double boiler and heat until warm. Apply to skin, avoiding the eyes, and leave on for 15 minutes. Remove with warm, wet washcloth.

Banana Mask

Blend one medium or large banana until smooth. Apply to skin, avoiding the delicate eye area. Leave on 15 minutes, then remove with a warm, wet washcloth.

Bran-Yogurt Mask
For troubled skin

4 tablespoons finely ground bran flakes
1 tablespoon plain yogurt

Mix yogurt into the bran to form a thick paste. Smooth over skin. Wait 15 minutes, then rinse with warm water.

Brewer's Yeast Mask

2 tablespoons brewer's yeast
1 tablespoon mineral water
1 egg white

In a bowl, beat egg white until frothy. Add mineral water and beat again. Stir in brewer's yeast to form a thick paste. Stroke over skin with upward motions, avoiding the delicate skin around the eyes. Leave on for 20 minutes. Remove with warm, wet washcloth. Rinse face thoroughly with warm water.

Buttermilk Mask

1/4 cup oatmeal
Buttermilk

Grind the oatmeal in a blender or coffee grinder until powdery. Slowly add just enough buttermilk to form a thick paste. Apply to skin and leave on for 20 minutes. Rinse with warm water.

Camphor Mask
For troubled skin

1 egg white
1 teaspoon olive oil
1/4 teaspoon camphor

Beat the egg white slightly, then mix in olive oil and camphor. Using fingertips, spread the mixture over the skin and leave on 20 minutes. Rinse with warm water.

Cucumber Mask

1 peeled cucumber
1/4 teaspoon lemon juice
1 teaspoon witch hazel
1 teaspoon alcohol
1 egg white

Juice the cucumber. Add the liquid ingredients and stir well. In another bowl, beat the egg white until frothy, then add to cucumber mixture. Apply to skin and leave on for 20 or 30 minutes. Rinse well with warm water.

Herbal Home Sauna I

Boil six quarts of water. Remove from the heat and add one cup of the following, according to your skin type:

peppermint for oily skin, chamomile for normal skin, or rosemary for dry skin. Let it steep for five minutes. Protect eyes, lips and hairline with petroleum jelly, then drape a large towel over your head and the pot, and let the vapors bathe your face for about ten minutes. Caution: Don't get too close to the pot as the steam can burn. Hold your head about 12 to 16 inches away from the pot. When you are finished, gently blot your skin with a soft, fluffy towel and apply toner and moisturizer.

Herbal Home Sauna II

Boil six quarts of water. Remove from heat and add 1 cup of fennel seeds. Steep for five minutes. Follow directions above for protecting the face and steaming. When finished, take a small amount of the water, about a quarter cup; strain any fennel from it. Add enough honey to make a paste and apply to the face and lie down for 20 minutes while it penetrates the skin. Remove with a warm, wet washcloth and apply moisturizer.

Honey Mask I

1 egg yolk
1 tablespoon honey
1 teaspoon olive oil

Beat the egg yolk into the oil thoroughly, then add the honey. Apply to the face with your fingertips. Leave on for 15 minutes, then rinse thoroughly with warm water.

Honey Mask II

1 whole egg
1 tablespoon honey

Whip the egg until frothy; mix in honey. Apply to skin and leave on for 20 minutes. Rinse with warm water, then follow with cool water.

Honey and Oatmeal Mask

2 tablespoons finely ground oatmeal
1 ounce honey
1 teaspoon lemon juice
1/2 teaspoon oil of sweet almonds
2 unbeaten egg whites

In a bowl, mix honey, lemon juice, almond oil and egg whites. When smooth, slowly add the oatmeal until it forms a paste. Spread over the skin and leave on for 20 minutes. Rinse with warm water.

Milk Mask

1 package dry milk powder
Buttermilk

Mix enough buttermilk into dry milk powder to make a thick paste. Apply to skin and leave on for 20 minutes. Rinse with warm water.

Oatmeal Mask

1/2 cup milk
2 tablespoons unprocessed oatmeal
2 teaspoons elder flower water

Prepare oatmeal according to package directions, using milk in place of water. Remove from heat and add the elder flower water. Stir thoroughly. Let mixture cool until it is warm but not hot. Apply to skin; leave on for 20 minutes. Remove with warm water, rinsing thoroughly.

Olive Oil Mask

1 cup olive oil
1 egg
2 tablespoons lemon juice
1/2 teaspoon sea salt

Blend half the oil with the remaining ingredients. Whip until it thickens, then pour in the remaining oil very slowly, beating continuously. Apply to face and leave on for 15 to 30 minutes. Rinse with warm water. Store any remainder in the refrigerator.

Parsley Facial

1 cup distilled water
1 tablespoon honey
1 egg yolk
1/2 cup parsley

Boil the parsley in the water for 15 minutes, then strain and allow to cool. Beat the egg yolk and stir in the honey, then combine with the parsley liquid, mixing thoroughly. Apply to face and leave on for 15 minutes. Rinse with warm water.

Wheat Germ Facial

3/4 cup oil of sweet almonds
1 teaspoon distilled water
1/2 teaspoon wheatgerm
1 egg yolk

Beat the egg yolk and almond oil together, then add the water and beat again until smooth. Finally, add the wheat germ. Apply to the face and leave on 20 minutes. Remove with warm, wet washcloth and rinse thoroughly.

Yeast Mask

2 tablespoons brewer's yeast
2 tablespoons skim milk

Add the milk to the brewer's yeast and mix until it forms a paste. Spread evenly over the face, avoiding the eye area, and leave on for 10 minutes. Remove with warm, wet washcloth, then rinse thoroughly with warm water.

Yogurt Mask

1/2 cup plain yogurt
1 tablespoon calcium carbonate

Mix the calcium carbonate into the yogurt, beating until it reaches a smooth, creamy consistency. Smooth over the face, avoiding the eye area, and leave on 10 to 15 minutes. Rinse thoroughly with warm water.

SKIN PREPARATIONS
--- FOR SPECIAL PROBLEMS ---

Blackhead Lotion

1 tablespoon Epsom salts
1 cup boiling water
3 drops white iodine

Dissolve Epsom salts and iodine in boiling water. Let cool slightly. Saturate a cotton pad and apply to the face while still hot, but not boiling. This will soften the blackheads so they can be easily removed.

Blackhead Remover

4 ounces ground almonds
3 ounces powdered oatmeal

2 ounces powdered orris root
1/2 ounce grated castile soap
2 tablespoons water

Thoroughly mix the dry ingredients together. Stir the water into the dry ingredients to make a paste. Rub onto blackheads and leave on one hour. Remove with a warm, wet washcloth and rinse thoroughly.

Blemish Lotion

1 ounce powdered alum
1 ounce lemon juice
1 pint rose water

Combine all the ingredients in a bottle and refrigerate. Shake thoroughly before using. To use, saturate a cotton pad with the lotion and gently swab over the troubled areas. Leave on overnight.

Blemish Cream I

2 pints rose water
2 finely chopped apples
2 tablespoons chopped fennel
2 tablespoons chopped celery
1 teaspoon lanolin
1/4 ounce barley meal
3 egg whites

Simmer the rose water, apples, fennel, celery and barley meal in a double boiler until they turn to mush. In a bowl, beat egg whites until frothy, then slowly add the lanolin to the egg whites. Combine egg white mixture with rose water mixture. Strain, then beat until smooth. Apply to affected skin areas as needed. Store remainder in refrigerator between uses.

Blemish Cream II

1 tablespoon castor oil
1 tablespoon glycerine
1 tablespoon lanolin

Place all ingredients in the top of a double boiler and heat until melted. Remove from heat, cool, and store in a glass jar. Use as needed.

Freckle Fading Cream I

1/4 cup sour milk
1/2 teaspoon grated horseradish
1 tablespoon cornmeal or powdered oatmeal

Combine all ingredients, forming a paste. Put between two layers of gauze, then apply to freckled areas, avoiding the eyes. Leave for 30 minutes, then remove with warm, wet washcloth and rinse thoroughly. Refrigerate any remaining cream.

Freckle Fading Cream II

3 tablespoons distilled water
3 teaspoons lemon juice
1/4 teaspoon cream of tartar
1/4 ounce oil of bitter almonds
1 ounce grated castile soap
4 drops olive oil

Melt the grated soap and water in a double boiler over low heat. When water has evaporated, mix in the rest of the ingredients. Blend thoroughly. Rub gently over the freckles and leave on skin for 30 minutes. Remove with warm, wet washcloth, and rinse thoroughly. Refrigerate remainder.

GLYCOLIC ACID

Chances are you've heard about the exciting, wrinkle-reducing results delivered by Retin-A. But you may not be aware that many people have several side effects from Retin-A use, including redness, rashes and peeling. Virtually any amount of sun exposure can exacerbate these effects. And people with sensitive skin dislike the stinging sensation it causes.

A milder compound called glycolic acid has been discovered to provide the same benefits with fewer side effects. Research shows that this acid, which is derived from sugar cane and is one of a class of compounds known as alpha-hydroxy acids, helps the skin slough the dead surface cells that accumulate on the skin's surface. It improves skin texture, evens out skin tone and also diminishes brown spots.

Recent test results show that it helps human fibroblast cells produce more collagen and elastin within as little as 24 hours. These collagen-rich new cells forming in the basal layer will begin to surface in as little as two weeks.

— MAKEUP MAGIC —

In the beginning of this book, you learned what happens to the skin as it ages: it becomes thinner as it loses underlying fat padding, less elastic due to a decrease in collagen, and more colorless as it loses pigmentation. This is where the magic of makeup combined with the art of proper application can help. Professional makeup artists know how to take five to ten years off your face in just minutes with a few little tricks using the principle of *trompe l'oeil*—fooling the eye.

Face Makeup

Use a light-textured foundation. Heavy foundations will mask the face and make you look older. Don't try to add color to your skin with your foundation; let your blusher fill that function. Instead, choose a neutral color as close to your natural skin tone as possible. Test the color on your cheek, not your wrist. No one wears makeup on their wrist! The color should seem to vanish into your own skin tone; if it doesn't blend into your skin, don't buy it. Keep looking until you find one that does. The ideal face makeup doesn't call attention to itself; instead, it prepares the face, like a blank canvas waiting for the artistic touch of color on cheeks, lips and eyes.

To apply, smooth the foundation gently over the skin with a slightly damp sponge, always using downward strokes. Or spritz the face lightly with mineral water or toner, then glide foundation on with fingertips over your dampened skin. When you are finished, spritz lightly again to set the foundation. Blend foundation carefully under the jaw and around the jawline, but don't extend it onto the neck where it will get onto your clothes.

MAGIC TRICK: A lavender color corrector used under your foundation will minimize broken capillaries.

Powder

After foundation, apply powder in this fashion: put a small amount of powder in the palm of your hand and dip a large, fluffy brush or cotton puff into it. Shake off excess, then dust the T-zone area of your face lightly, starting at the chin and working up. When finished, whisk away excess powder with a clean makeup brush. Use a very fine-textured, translucent loose powder with no color in it—any color in the powder will change the color of your foundation, and call attention to fine lines and wrinkles. Loose powder is preferable to compact powder, which is intended to be carried in the purse for a quick touch-up.

MAGIC TRICK: Don't powder your cheeks—it has a very aging effect. The glow on your cheeks will look naturally youthful.

Blusher

When selecting a blusher, stay in the same color family as your hair. A simple rule of thumb: Blondes should choose light, tawny tones; brunettes can go for rose, mauve or reddish-brown tones; redheads should use peach and coral tones. If your hair is grey, you may use clear rose or red tones. Apply blusher correctly; little round circles on the cheeks are for clowns, not beautiful women. To find out where to apply blusher, look in the mirror and smile. Next, place two fingers alongside your nose. Blusher should begin next to the finger farthest from your nose. Sweep blush up and out, toward the hairline. This has a "lifting" effect, and gives the illusion of pulling the face up.

MAGIC TRICK: Brush a deep mauve blusher along the jawline, from one to the other under the chin. This helps to conceal a double chin instantly and also gives the jawline a clearer, more sharply defined look.

Lips

As you get older, the natural line of the lip becomes less clearly defined and a lifetime of mouth movements can lead to fine vertical lines around the lips. Lipstick seeps or "bleeds" into these lines. Lipliner can help prevent this "bleeding" and keep lip color in place, as well as adding definition to the mouth. Lipliner also gives a cleaner, fresher look than lipstick alone. First, apply foundation to the lips and let dry. Then, use a lipliner to outline the lips with a thick line, starting with the bottom lip first, working from the center out. Extend slightly at the corner to give the mouth an upward lift. Then outline the upper lip, again working from the center out. Then fill in with lip color—either lipstick or lipliner.

You should not attempt to reshape the entire mouth, but with subtle application, lip color can minimize flaws. For a mouth that's too big, outline just inside the natural lipline with a light color and fill in with a deeper tone. For lips that are too full, use a lipliner in the same shade as your lipstick and avoid bright, shiny colors; keep lipstick just inside natural lipline. For lips that are too thin, outline in a light shade just outside the natural lipline, stopping a little short of the corners, and fill in with a deeper shade. For lips that are unequal in thickness, use a darker color for the thicker lip and a lighter color for the thinner one.

When choosing a lip color, stay in the same color family as your blusher. Stay away from pastels with white undertones, deep wine or burgundy colors, and especially fire-engine red. Colors that are very dramatic or too white will emphasize any wrinkles that you may have around the mouth area.

LIP LINES

Fine lines around the lips can be smoothed away using one tablespoon sea salt mixed into a cup of boiling mineral water. After the water has cooled, rub the saline solution gently over the fine lines on your upper lip.

Use this procedure twice weekly, and you'll see the lines begin to fade away, unless there is another underlying cause.

Dental problems, such as missing teeth and gum erosion, can cause fine lines around the lip as well as a sagging jawline and shrunken-looking mouth. Ask your dentist about reconstructive dentistry to correct any problems.

MAGIC TRICK: Apply a smidgeon of clear gloss in the center of the lower lip. This will draw the eye away from upper lip lines.

MAGIC TRICK: If your mouth droops at the corners, draw attention away by not extending your lip color all the way. When outlining the lips, stop short and draw the liner up. Fill in the rest of the mouth with lip color, also stopping short of the corners. Using a darker lip color on the bottom lip will help draw attention away from droopy lips, too.

Eyes

The eyes have been called windows to the soul. Along with the mouth, they are the main focus of the face. The following tips and techniques will draw attention to your beautiful, expressive eyes, not your wrinkles.

Eye Shadow: Always use a moisturizer on the upper eyelids as an undercoat before applying eye shadow. Be careful to use a light hand when applying eye makeup—the Cleopatra look has not been popular for quite a while. Use the principles of light and dark when choosing eye shadows. Remember that light colors highlight and dark colors recede. If your eyes are deep-set, a lighter shadow will draw them out. Use only pale translucent or matte eye shadows in soft, muted colors. Never use iridescent eye shadows—they will magnify every crease and line on the eyelid. If your eyelids are very lined, try using cream eye shadows rather than powder shadows, which can be very drying. Powder eye shadows will also get caught in any wrinkles you may have on your eyelids. Experts recommend choosing complementary eye shadows rather than coordinating them with your outfit.

MAGIC TRICK: If your eyelids are very wrinkled, use a dark foundation on the eyelids instead of eye shadow; it will give a dewy, natural look.

MAGIC TRICK: For a youthful, wide-eyed look, only use eye shadow on the outer half of your eyelids.

Eyeliner: Use brown eyeliner rather than black, which gives the eyes a hard-edged, older look, and choose a smudge stick rather than a hard stick, which will pull the delicate eye skin. To turn those old pencils into eye-friendly smudge sticks, light a match and hold the flame a few inches away from the tip for a few seconds. You don't want to melt the color, just soften it. After it has cooled, but before it returns to its previous hard state, you can use it to gently outline your eyes.

MAGIC TRICK: Use liner instead of shadows on very wrinkled lids. Line the eye with a dark brown or charcoal liner, and smudge with a soft brush. The liner should not be a hard line, which is aging; instead, it should look like the root of the lashes.

Eyelashes: The same caution about color applies to mascara—use a brown or a black-brown mascara for everyday wear and save the heavy, dramatic black mascara for those romantic, candlelit evenings, where the lighting is diffused.

MAGIC TRICK: To make eyes look wider and more open, curl your lashes then apply two coats of mascara on upper lashes and one light coat on the lower lashes. Too much mascara on the lower lashes is aging.

Eyebrows: Beautifully shaped eyebrows framing beautiful eyes can direct attention away from crow's-feet and tiny lines around the eye. But improperly cared-for eyebrows can compound any problems you may have, such as droopy eyes or crepey eyelids.

To determine the proper shape for your eyebrows, look in the mirror. The eyebrow should begin just above each side of the nose and end just at the outside corner of the eye. The arch should be slightly to the side of the pupil of the eye. You may have to do some tweezing to get the results you want. Follow these suggestions for shaping beautiful brows:

- Remove all eye makeup. Saturate a cotton ball with rubbing alcohol and squeeze out the excess. Gently wipe the ball along the arch of the brow to remove any remaining eye makeup remover.

- Soak a washcloth in very warm water, wring it out, and press over the eyebrows for a minute. The warmth will open the pores, making it easier to tweeze the hairs. If you are very sensitive, you can rub an ice cube over the area you're going to tweeze. It will numb the skin and reduce the pain.

- Begin tweezing the hairs growing between the brows, over the nose. Always tweeze in the direction the hair grows and only pull one hair at a time. Get as close to the base of the hair as possible, firmly grip the hair, and pull it out without hesitating.

- Tweeze any straggly hairs underneath to emphasize the arch. Only tweeze from the underside of the brows. *Never* tweeze from above; this is unnatural looking and it undermines the arch as well. Be careful when shaping: too-thin eyebrows are very aging because the eyebrow thins naturally as you get older. And nothing is more aging than penciled-in eyebrows. To thin bushy brows: Brush the hairs down, then trim along the natural arch with manicure scissors. Brush up and out when finished.

MAGIC TRICK: Shorten the outer end of the eyebrow for an upswept, winged look that will lift the entire face.

When applying brow makeup, choose a color one shade

lighter than your hair color. If your hair is grey, your brows should be one shade darker than your hair. You can have your eyebrows lightened at a salon, or do them at home with a safe, facial-hair bleach. You can darken them with a light brown or taupe pencil. Never use dark brown or black eyebrow pencils or makeup; it's too harsh.

MAGIC TRICK: For an instant eyelift, spritz a little hair fixative or put a dab of hair gel or moustache wax on an eyebrow brush or toothbrush and brush brows up.

To Minimize Dark Circles: After cleansing and moisturizing the face, use a color-correcting underbase before applying foundation. To minimize blue circles, use a pale yellow underbase. Use a pale blue or mauve underbase to minimize brown circles. Use these color correctors only on the undereye area. Never use a white or very light concealer to hide circles.

To Make Tired Eyes Look Brighter: First, use eye drops formulated for allergy and cold symptoms to help clear the red up fast. While you're waiting for the eyedrops to work, try placing a washcloth dampened with cool water; chilled cucumber or potato slices, or cold, damp tea bags on your eyelids. Wait five minutes then remove. Your eyes will feel refreshed. Use a blue liner to make the whites of the eyes appear brighter. Try using blue mascara on the tips of the upper lashes, applied over your usual mascara. Stay away from heavy, dark shadows, which will only make eyes look older and more tired. To make eyes look fresher and clearer, place a dot of concealer just under the arch of the eyebrow and blend.

To Minimize Fine Lines and Crow's-Feet: To camouflage crow's-feet and fine lines under the eye, use an undereye concealer *over*, not under, the foundation. Use a shade close to your own skin tone; do not use white, which will emphasize the lines rather than conceal them. Don't apply eye shadow beyond the eyelid; it will draw attention to crow's-feet.

— BATHING BEAUTY—

Through the ages, many famous beauties have used their baths as rejuvenating spas. You can do the same. The addition of scented oils and skin softeners to the bath helps prevent the skin from getting rough and flaky by replacing lost moisture and oil. Fragrant herbs in the bath can turn it into a soothing and healing, or invigorating and energizing experience, depending on the herbs and water temperature.

Temperature

The temperature of the water will determine whether your bath is a relaxing or a revitalizing one. Test the water with the inside of your wrist or your elbow, or use a thermometer if desired. Extreme temperatures are not recommended for anyone, but anyone with poor circulation should be especially wary of extremely hot or cold water. Water over 100 degrees Fahrenheit should not be used as it can cause the surface veins in the legs to break. Also, extremely hot water can strip the skin of its acid mantle, dehydrating the skin.

Warm: 85 to 100 degrees Fahrenheit is the best temperature for a relaxing bath. As relaxing as a nice warm tub is, don't stay in too long—no longer than 20 minutes. Overhydration is as bad for your skin as dehydration; after 20 minutes, the skin begins to shrivel, becoming prune-like, which is only attractive to another prune.

RELAXING RITUAL

Create your own personal bath ritual. Run the tub full of warm water and add one of the scented oils or fragrant herbs listed. The delicately scented water will calm your nerves while soothing and pampering your skin by adding moisture and replenishing the precious skin oils lost during the day. The warmth of the bathwater relaxes the muscles and relieves tension by temporarily lowering the blood pressure.

Make your bathing ritual even more special: turn the lights down low, light a special candle and use the time to meditate. Splurge on some extra thick, fluffy towels and use them to gently blot the excess moisture from your skin when you step out of the tub. Never rub your skin dry; always be gentle with your skin. Leave skin slightly damp and apply a scented body moisturizer or lotion all over your body. The gentle scent will promote soothing, peaceful sleep.

Use a loofah in bath and shower for all-over body sloughing. *Caution:* Be sure to hang the loofah to dry. Once a week, soak it for a few minutes in a two-percent bleach solution. This will help avoid skin infections by killing any microorganisms that may be lurking in your loofah.

Tepid: 75 to 85 degrees Fahrenheit will revive and

refresh you during hot weather. Taking a bath at this temperature for 10 to 15 minutes can help you stay cool for several hours afterward. It gives the circulatory system the opportunity to release internal heat through the skin.

Cool: 65 to 75 degrees Fahrenheit is the ideal temperature for a quick jump-start at the beginning of the day or as a pick-me-up after work. Don't stay in the tub longer than 10 minutes at this temperature.

Cold: 65 degrees Fahrenheit or less is an instant eye-opener. Water at this temperature is very stimulating, and gives the blood circulation a real boost. The best way to approach it is by plunging in quickly and getting out immediately. If it is too difficult to get into a tub of water at this temperature, try taking a shower with the water pressure on high. You'll instantly feel invigorated and refreshed.

There are basically three types of baths: soothing, stimulating and restoring. Following a discussion of the different types of baths are some recipes you can make using common ingredients found in most kitchens. There is also a partial listing of essential oils and their properties that you can add to your bath to make it even more rewarding.

Soothing Baths

These baths will soften the skin and combat dryness. You may use cool water but warm is more soothing.

- **Milk:** Add a cup of powdered milk to a warm bath for a modern version of Cleopatra's fabled milk bath.

- **Oatmeal:** Add one pound of oatmeal to a warm

bath. The oils in oatmeal will smooth and nourish the skin. Be sure to rinse thoroughly before toweling off. You can also make a scrub bag to use in the tub. Combine one pound of oatmeal, four ounces bran flour, four ounces powdered orris root (available at health food stores) with one bar of finely shredded castile soap and place in a bag made of muslin or cheesecloth. You may substitute almond meal for the oatmeal. Place this bag in your bath mitt or in another bag made of terry cloth. Use either as a bath mitt, rubbing it over the skin, or throw it into the bath water and let it soak like a teabag. It will last through several baths.

- **Milk and Honey:** Dissolve two ounces bicarbonate of soda and four ounces sea salt in a pint of lukewarm water. Warm three pints of milk (you can use dried milk, reconstituting according to package directions), and add one pound honey. Pour the soda-and-salt mixture into the bath, then add the milk and honey, and relax.

- **Starch:** The addition of two teaspoons of ordinary laundry starch will soften even the hardest water, as well as smoothing the skin.

Stimulating

Mineral salts added to the bath will stimulate the circulatory system, help eliminate toxins and refresh the skin. You'll feel invigorated by their addition to either a warm or cool bath.

- **Seaweed:** Fill a muslin or cheesecloth bag with seaweed and toss it in the bath about 10 minutes before you get in. Turns your bathtub into your own personal sea resort.

- **Sea Salt**: An excellent exfoliator. You can rub a handful or two of sea salt over the body, avoiding the face, or put the salt in a cloth bag or bath mitt.

- **Epsom Salts:** For a wonderfully therapeutic bath, add eight ounces of epsom salts to a warm bath. To enhance the benefits of this bath, add mint or eucalyptus oils.

Restoring

You can get the benefit of spa-type bath treatments in the comfort of your own home without paying a fortune at a private health resort. You should always use warm water for these baths, which are soothing before bedtime or ideal for relaxing after work.

- **Herbal:** To use, put the herbs in a muslin or cheesecloth bag or make an infusion to add to the bath water. Don't just throw the herbs in the bath; they can clog the drains and are difficult to clean out of the tub and off yourself. To make an infusion, place two teaspoons of herbs into a pot and add one pint of boiling water. Cover pot and let steep for at least 15 minutes. The longer the herb steeps, the more effective it will be, up to a maximum of three hours. Don't limit yourself to a single herb; be creative and make your own mixtures, or use the following herbal combinations. See the list of herbal properties under "Essential Oils" to spark your imagination; the herbs have the same properties as the oils.

- **Lavender:** Mix dried lavender flowers with mint leaves and rosemary.

- **Rosemary:** Mix equal amounts of rosemary, fennel, sage, and yarrow.

- **Chamomile:** Add rosemary and pine needles to either fresh or dried chamomile flowers.

- **Blackberry Tonic:** Make a strong infusion and add to warm bath to restore a dull skin.

- **Pine Needles:** Boil for 20 minutes, then steep for 12 hours. Strain and add one cupful to bath. Store the remainder in the refrigerator for later use.

- **Cider Vinegar:** Vinegar will restore the skin's acid mantle. Add one cupful to the bath.

Essential Oils for the Bath

Essential oils make a wonderful addition to the bath. Because they are extremely concentrated, only a drop or two is necessary. The list below gives the traditional uses of these oils. Get one of the many books on aromatherapy for more information and other uses of these oils.

- **Anise** stimulates circulation and respiration.

- **Basil** clarifies the mental processes.

- **Bergamot** is used to treat depression.

- **Camphor** is used as both a congestion clearing inhalant and a muscle liniment.

- **Chamomile** contains azulene, which is very

soothing to the skin. It is also used to treat stress, irritability, depression, and migraines because it is calming and refreshing.

- **Elder** is calming and restoring. It also has healing properties and stimulates the skin.

- **Eucalyptus** is an excellent decongestant, widely used as an inhalant for colds and fevers.

- **Geranium** has a calming effect.

- **Jasmine** has a soothing effect on the nerves.

- **Lavender** relaxes both the nervous system and the muscular system; helps encourage a calm and peaceful disposition.

- **Lemon** invigorates the skin.

- **Marjoram** is a natural sedative and has a tranquilizing effect.

- **Melissa** has antiseptic qualities and is used as an antidepressant and to calm nervous tension.

- **Mint** is stimulating and energizing.

- **Orange** is cheerful and uplifting.

- **Rose** is soothing and calming, good for anxiety, depression and circulatory problems.

- **Rosemary** is called the memory herb for its stimulating effect on mental faculties.

- **Sage** makes a relaxing, warming bath, producing feelings of euphoric well being.

- **Sandalwood** is relaxing, promoting tranquility.

- **Spearmint** refreshes muscles.

- **Tea tree** has many uses. It is a powerful antiseptic, destroying harmful bacteria and preserv-
  ing healthy tissue. Promotes faster healing.

- **Thyme** is mentally and physically fortifying.

- **Ylang Ylang** is emotionally soothing, has a euphoric effect, and arouses physical energies.

— SLEEP —

Sleep is as important to a beautiful complexion as good
nutrition, proper skin care and moisture. Chronic skimping
on sleep can turn fine lines into furrows. Remember that
your body uses the sleeping hours to regenerate the body—
metabolizing nutrients and eliminating wastes—so help
your body heal itself by giving it the sleep it needs, and
following these tips:

- **Learn correct sleeping posture.** Pushing your
  face into a pillow night after night can lead to
  permanent wrinkles. It may take some time, but
  you can retrain yourself to sleep on your back.
  If you prefer sleeping on your side, turn your
  face to a 45-degree angle to avoid pillow lines.
  Many chiropractors recommend the use of a
  neck-roll pillow for proper neck alignment.
  Sprinkle a few drops of a soothing essential oil
  on a cotton pad and tuck it into the pillowcase.

- **Follow your skin regime before retiring.** Never
  go to bed with stale makeup on. Be sure you
  have scrupulously cleaned and moisturized your

skin. If the air is dry, use a humidifier.

- **Avoid morning face.** Nighttime fluid retention can cause morning puffiness. One solution is to cut down salt and alcohol intake, and don't drink too many fluids right before bedtime. Another solution is to elevate your head while sleeping. This improves circulation and keeps body fluids from collecting in your face.

Hair—Your Crowning Glory

A beautiful, shining head of hair can be your crowning glory but if your tresses are dull, dry or damaged, they can signal your age long before any wrinkles mar your features. Because hair color fades with age, those shining locks that were your pride and joy may need a refresher course.

Before you decide to brighten dull, age-faded color or cover grey, be sure that your hair is in tip-top condition. Nothing looks worse than a head full of brightly colored, straw-like hair.

—HAIR CARE—

Hair becomes thinner and finer with age, as well as losing pigment. After about age thirty, hair becomes duller, less shiny. Hair is composed of cells layered on top of each other, like the scales on a fish. When those cells lie flat, they reflect light. When hair is dirty or damaged, the cells lift, deflecting light rather than reflecting it. Daily washing with a moisturizing shampoo can help dry hair, which is caused by lack of moisture, not lack of oil. Consumer magazines say that advances in science and technology have greatly improved conditioners and shampoos in the last twenty years, so experiment with different products. Or ask your hairdresser to recommend a line of hair-care products to improve your hair's particular problems. Switch products every four to six months, since hair adjusts to any product after a period of time and no longer responds to it. Also, your hair care needs change with the seasons. Hair is drier and more flyaway during winter months, so choose a shampoo containing polyquaternium-10, which will help control static electricity. During summer months, when the hair is exposed to more sunlight and harsh chlorine or saltwater, use a shampoo fortified with sunscreen. If you color your hair or use other permanent processes, such as perming or straightening your hair, be sure to use shampoos and conditioners formulated for these conditions.

Before washing your hair, brush gently to remove dead hairs. Use a natural bristle brush to avoid breakage, and begin brushing at the nape of the neck, working up. Be sure to clean the brush weekly by soaking in ammonia and water, rinse and let dry. Next, massage the scalp, using a gentle kneading motion. Wet hair thoroughly with warm water. Pour a small amount of shampoo into the palm of your hand and work into a lather before applying to hair. Massage the lather gently through the hair with the balls of your fingers; no rubbing or scrubbing. Finally, rinse with warm water. If your hair is very oily or dirty, you may need to repeat the process a second time, but it's usually unnecessary. This is an additional step that was designed to increase product use, resulting in more product sales and higher profits for the manufacturer.

—SCALP—

Don't neglect the scalp when caring for your hair. The follicles are nourished by the scalp. Regular massage can give you a healthier head of hair by improving the scalp's circulation and blood supply. The ideal time to massage the scalp is either just before or during shampooing. The proper way to massage the scalp is to gently move the skin, using a circular movement. Start at the hairline and work toward the back. Don't scrub or rub the scalp; as you massage, you should feel the skin moving on the skull bone.

—THINNING HAIR—

Women can suffer from thinning hair as well as men. This can be caused by an increase in hormone production, which occurs after giving birth, or in response to increased responsibilities and tensions. It can also be caused by anxiety, worry, lack of sleep, and low protein intake. Continually pulling the hair back with a rubber band can cause hair to break off and cause inflammation of the scalp, leading to hair loss.

Some women may qualify to use minoxidil to encourage hair growth. It should be noted that any sudden or extreme hair loss should be reported to a physician for an appropriate medical evaluation as this may be a symptom of a more serious problem.

— HAIR COLOR—

Hair color comes from the pigment in the hair shaft. As you age, the pigmented hair strands are replaced by non-pigmented (grey or white) strands. When you think about coloring your hair, remember that your skin texture and tone has changed since you were young. As your skin changes color, Nature has replaced the vibrant hair colors of your youth with a more skin-flattering lighter tone. Keep this in mind when deciding to color grey or white hair. Don't opt for the same intensity of color you had when young; instead, choose a hair color a few shades lighter than your own original color. Too-dark hair color looks artificial and emphasizes age lines and skin imperfections.

Choose one of the new, longer-lasting semi-permanent hair colors available rather than a permanent hair color. Because they do not bleach the hair shaft, they cause less damage to your hair. Another bonus is that they don't look as artificial as monochromatic hair dyes. They blend with your hair, minimizing the difference between pigmented and gray strands.

For a totally natural haircolor without chemicals, consider using henna. Perform a strand test before applying to the total head as color stabilization may be difficult. Be sure to shampoo hair before application to ensure even color distribution. Follow package directions and be prepared to spend at least four hours or longer on the total process, depending on the results you want.

To add a brown tone to grey hair, make a strong infusion of sage and black tea. Boil the herbs for 30 minutes, then let it steep for three or four hours. Strain and apply to the grey hairs daily until they attain the desired shade. For a reddish tone, use saffron or marigold flowers. Prepare the flowers as an infusion, then use the liquid as a rinse, catching it in a basin and repeating the process many times.

For a quick color touch-up abetween tintings, dark hair colors can use cake eyeliner applied with an eyebrow brush. Wet the brush and rub over the cake eyeliner, then apply to any grey showing around the hairline.

— CUT —

The proper cut can create an optical illusion, manipulating light, color and shadow to beautifully frame your face. Generally speaking, older women need more height in their hair cuts to counteract the overall dropping effect gravity has on the face. Long flowing hair may have suited you perfectly as a teenager, but consider going shorter or adding volume to attract attention away from feature flaws.

An artfully cut fringe of bangs will pull the focus to your beautiful, expressive eyes and away from a pointy or receding chin. Making the hair slightly lighter around the face will minimize under-eye bags.

Positioning the most dramatic highlights just above the temple lifts the eye area. Hairstyles that sweep up at the sides also help lift the face, making it seem more youthful.

Draw attention away from a drooping jawline by darkening the hair at the lower sides and lightening the bangs or hair at the crown. Avoid blunt, chin-length cuts, which emphasize the jawline.

HOME REMEDIES FOR
—DRY HAIR—

Use these time-honored recipes, containing ingredients found in most refrigerators, to provide a quick, inexpensive assist to dry, damaged hair.

Mayonnaise Conditioner

Measure about one-quarter cup of mayonnaise (use real mayonnaise containing egg, not the cholesterol-free variety). Wet hair thoroughly with warm water. Blot hair with towel, then apply the mayonnaise evenly throughout the hair, paying special attention to drier ends. Cover hair with plastic cap (the kind used for coloring hair is fine) or dip the towel in warm water, wring it out and wrap it around your head turban-style. Relax for 15 to 30 minutes, then step into the shower and rinse hair thoroughly. Shampoo and follow with the rest of your daily hair ritual.

Protein Hair Restorer

Beat together 2 eggs. While beating, slowly add 1 tablespoon olive oil, 1 tablespoon glycerine and 1 teaspoon cider vinegar. After shampooing and rinsing hair, blot excess moisture from hair and apply. Leave on for 20 to 30 minutes, then rinse well.

Egg and Yogurt Conditioner

Measure out three or four tablespoons of plain yogurt. Break an egg into the yogurt and mix thoroughly. Following the steps above for wetting the hair, then apply the yogurt and egg mixture to hair, paying special attention to the drier ends. Cover hair with plastic cap or warm, damp towel.

Relax for 15 to 30 minutes, then rinse hair thoroughly.

Natural Highlighting Conditioners

To add subtle highlights and extra body to your hair, add the following to four ounces of olive oil: For highlights in dark hair, add 1/2 teaspoon each of rosemary and lavender oils. For light hair, add 1/2 teaspoon each of lavender, chamomile and lemon oils. Apply sparingly at night to scalp and hair. Wash hair thoroughly in the morning. Store any remaining mixture in the refrigerator.

The Rest of You

The final step in projecting an aura of youthful vitality is recapturing the lean, firm body you had when you were younger. Or, if you weren't lean and firm as a youth, developing a new, sleek image. It's never too late to develop good habits that can help keep you young and fit well into what were once considered the declining years.

Youthful looks are synonymous with beauty; the basis of all beauty is a healthy body. And a healthy body is dependent upon good diet, proper nutrition and exercise. Check with your local library or bookstore and pick up one of the many excellent books available on diet, nutrition and exercise.

— EXERCISE—

Exercise can help you regain the vigor and vitality you thought you had lost by boosting muscular strength and aerobic endurance. In fact, experts say that improving the quality of life is the number one motivator for exercise, number two is to get in shape and prevent illness, and number three is the desire to improve the appearance. Be sure to check with your physician before beginning any exercise program.

WRINKLE WORKOUT

These exercises can help reduce or eliminate some of the more common wrinkles. They can be done while reading, watching television, even while commuting, if you don't mind an audience.

Flabby jowls: To smooth and tighten a flabby jawline, tilt your head back and let your mouth fall open naturally. Close your mouth slowly and hold for ten seconds. Feel the pull in the neck muscles. Repeat five times.

Upper-lip lines: Make faces like a fish. Pucker your lips, then pull your upper lip over the teeth. Alternate several times.

Smile lines: As character lines, they're fine, but deeply etched trenches are aging. Puff your cheeks out, à la Dizzy Gillespie blowing the horn. Release the air slowly and repeat several times.

Experts are showing that the biological markers of age can not only be stopped, they can be reversed. Two of these biomarkers—muscle strength and lean body mass—are significantly affected by exercise. If you don't exercise regularly, you lose about six pounds of muscle a decade, which is replaced by fat. Other biomarkers include blood pressure, cholesterol levels and your BMR—basal metabolic rate, the rate at which you burn off calories.

It has been widely recognized for many years throughout the medical community that prolonged inactivity leads to slower responses and lessened aerobic capacity. New studies are showing that three weeks of enforced inactivity is equivalent to almost 20 years of aging. Many of the bodily changes blamed on the aging process are really caused by a lack of activity. Physiological functions decay following insufficient exercise at any age. The proportion of lean body mass declines while fat increases; the body's ability to efficiently use oxygen drops; the body produces fewer red blood cells, lowering the immune response; there is an increased tendency toward heart disease from rising blood cholesterol and triglycerides as well as an increase in blood clotting; bones lose calcium, becoming thinner and more brittle. All these biomarkers of age can be stopped and reversed by devising and using a sensible plan of exercise.

Some tips to help you with your exercise plan:

- **Be realistic**. Don't expect to overcome a life-long aversion to exercise in a week or two. Don't be discouraged—you should start seeing results within two to three weeks from your exercise plan. Allow about three months to really get in the groove.

- **Set appropriate goals.** Have a lithe, healthy body as your goal, not a walking skeleton. Stringy muscles overlaying the bones are neither youthful looking nor attractive. Sharply protruding bones are as aging as flabby muscle tone and a roll around the middle.

- **Balance your exercise.** Do an aerobic exercise, such as walking, running or bicycling, for cardiovascular fitness, at least four times a week. Supplement your aerobic exercise with mild resistance training (weight training) two or three times a week. Once you have attained the level of fitness you desire, maintain that level by exercising a minimum of three times a week.

- **Focus your training.** Target the major muscle groups of the body; work one section one day, the rest in the next workout. For example, do upper body training on alternate days from lower body training.

- **Warm up and cool down.** Be sure to do stretching exercises after warming up to improve flexibility and prevent injury.

- **Set a schedule.** The biggest factor in the success of any exercise program is scheduling the time to do it and then sticking to your schedule. Be practical and choose times that are convenient and won't interfere with work or other responsibilities.

- **Use the buddy system.** If you hate to exercise alone, invite a friend to join your workouts. Peer pressure is a marvelous motivator and can make exercise more enjoyable.

- **Rest.** Overtraining your muscles can be as bad as undertraining or no training at all. Be sure to set aside one or two days a week to give your muscles a chance to recuperate from the stress of training.

EXERCISE CAN PREVENT CANCER

Several years ago, the Harvard Alumni Health Study, begun in the 1960s, proved that people who exercised tended to live longer lives. Now it is showing that those longer lives are healthier lives. The study found that people who burned 1,000 or more calories through exercise every week had half the risk of developing colon cancer as those who exercised less or not at all. 1,000 calories is the equivalent of walking ten miles or jogging for two hours. There are also some indications, unconfirmed as yet, that increased exercise may protect against prostate cancer.

— DIET AND NUTRITION —

You are what you eat. The kinds of food and nutrients you eat will determine the healthy, youthful appearance of hair, skin and body. You can color and shape your hair, apply concealing makeup skillfully and sculpt your body with exercise, but if you are inadequately fueling yourself with a poor-quality diet, the rest of your efforts will not accomplish much.

Because the immune system declines as we age, we become more susceptible to bacterial and viral infections as well as increasingly at risk for the degenerative diseases, such as cancer, arthritis and heart disease.

Including the right kinds of oils in your diet can not only help improve the health of your cardiovascular system, but add a healthy sheen to your skin as well. The easy way to do this is to take two 10-gram capsules of ecosapentaenoic acid (EPA or fish oil) and two 10-gram capsules of Evening Primrose oil daily.

Certain nutrients, such as vitamin B6 and the antioxidants beta-carotene and vitamins E and C, can help you to avoid, slow or reverse these supposedly inevitable symptoms of aging, especially of the immune system.

Antioxidants help prevent damage from chemicals called free radicals, which attack the body's cells and cause them to break down. Free radicals are caused by exposure to sunlight, pollution, cigarette smoke, certain drugs, and alcohol. They damage the collagen and elastin in the skin, and contribute to the formation of age spots by affecting the production of melanin, the skin-coloring pigment.

MAGIC MINERALS

Recent research shows that two minerals—molybdenum and magnesium—may have a profound effect on aging skin. A recommended dosage for noticeable skin improvement is 500 micrograms of molybdenum once a day, and magnesium (in the form of milk of magnesia tablets) three times a day.

Eat foods that contain the greatest amount of nutrients with the least amount of calories and fat: fresh fruits and vegetables, whole grains, lean meat, fish and poultry, and non-fat dairy products. A good anti-aging diet is one that incorporates the following principles:

- Decrease fat consumption to less than 30 percent of your total calorie intake. Shoot for a percentage between 15 to 25; experts say a diet with less than 15 percent fat is too flavorless for most people to stick with.

- Increase your fiber intake, getting at least 20 to 35 grams per day.

- Eat antioxidant-rich foods—those containing large amounts of vitamins E and C and beta-carotene (see recommended foods below).

- Maintain an adequate intake of calcium to prevent osteoporosis.

- Take a vitamin/mineral supplement to ensure adequate intake of necessary micronutrients.

- Store foods in airtight containers and avoid light exposure that may destroy valuable nutrients.

Beta-Carotene

Vegetables: Carrots, winter squash, pumpkin, sweet potatoes, and dark green vegetables, such as spinach and broccoli. **Fruits:** Apricots, cantaloupe, mangoes and peaches

Vitamin C

Vegetables: Red and green peppers, sweet potatoes, tomatoes, white potatoes, and cruciferous vegetables, such as broccoli, brussels sprouts, and cauliflower. **Fruits:** Citrus fruits (and juices), strawberries, and melons—honeydew, cantaloupe and watermelon.

Vitamin E

Vegetables: Green leafy vegetables, corn, and vegetable oils. **Other sources:** Nuts and seeds—sunflower seeds, filberts, almonds, peanut butter, soybeans and wheat germ.

Vitamin B6

Sources: Poultry, fish, lean pork, eggs. Peanuts, walnuts, soy beans, oats and whole-grain rice are other good sources.

HEALING THYME

Recent studies have scientists looking at the ability of the herb thyme to protect organs from damaging free-radicals. Tests on the livers of laboratory animals fed highly concentrated doses of the herb showed they had increased levels of polyunsaturated fatty acids. These acids, which help maintain the integrity of cell membranes, are especially susceptible to damage from free-radicals. Further testing could produce anti-aging drugs containing thyme in the future.

REJUVENATING THE INNER YOU

Inner Reality

You can color and shape your hair to a perfect, flattering frame, improve skin texture and tone and conceal minor facial flaws through skillful makeup application, and redefine your body with proper diet, nutrition and muscle-toning and sculpting exercise, but one of the most important ingredients to projecting a youthful image is an internal sense of balance and harmony. As the old saying goes, you are only as young as you think you are. Your mind is the computer that controls the biological processes that age you. You can reprogram that computer to slow down the aging process.

Think of all the people you've known who are youthful despite their age. More than any other factor, they have a zest for life, a continuing sense of wonder and curiosity, and an interest in the world around them. This mental agility, combined with a sense of peace and harmony, enables them to project a youthful exuberance and vitality that is forever young.

The Psychology of Aging

...

Feeling fit in mind as well as body will create a mental attitude, an excitement for life, that will make you feel young. You'll experience a state of robust good health, and the better you feel emotionally and physically, the younger you'll feel, no matter what your age.

Psychologist Abraham Maslow believed that, after they achieve their basic biological needs of food, water and shelter from danger and the elements, healthy people seek not only affection and self-respect but personal fulfillment, or what he called self-actualization.

These self-actualizing people exhibit more creativity, display a playful sense of humor, and have better interpersonal relationships. A person who has a sense of personal fulfillment is free to focus attention on such abstract concepts as justice, beauty, and understanding.

Food for Thought

It may seem contradictory to begin a section on the effect of the emotions, mind and attitude by discussing a purely physical subject like the diet. But the simple truth is that you can start being healthier and slowing down the aging process right now just by eating the right foods.

Our mind is the interface between the physical world and the non-physical. Even though our thoughts and feelings do not belong to the physical realm, they are influenced by that interface.

Because the brain is physical as well as mental, a healthy, youthfully functioning brain plays a key role in how you feel about yourself and the world around you. You can recharge, restore and rejuvenate your brain by giving it adequate nutritional support—micronutrients, vitamins, minerals and amino acids—and protecting it against the ravages of accumulated toxins like heavy metals.

The final step in ensuring a razor-sharp intellect and memory is to work the brain muscle with mental exercises. Your thinking will become clearer, your attitude will improve and you will have more energy. You will begin to not only feel younger, but to look and act younger.

— B-COMPLEX VITAMINS—

Vitamins are critical to healthy brain functioning, and play a key role in the brain's performance. The brain seems to have a special need for the B vitamins. They have been found to protect against mental slowness, memory defects, and mood disorders. Studies show that deficiencies of B vitamins may impair recent memory, produce depression, create apprehension, hyper-irritability, and emotional instability—deficiencies appearing more and more commonly in our modern urbanized society than ever before, to a large extent among the older population of Americans.

FEEDING YOUR HEAD

Brain performance can be regulated not only by what you eat but when you eat it. Post-meal drowsiness is caused by serotonin, a neurotransmitter that the brain synthesizes from the amino acid tryptophan. A high-carbohydrate meal causes the pancreas to secrete insulin, a hormone that encourages the muscles to pick up amino acids from the blood. More tryptophan enters the brain, which then produces more serotonin. Serotonin inhibits the electrical transmission between the neurons and induces sleep.

This is fine when you want to feel drowsy, relaxed and ready for bed, but if you want your neurons firing on all cylinders, keep carbohydrate intake at breakfast and lunch to a minimum. Emphasize protein; it helps keep the brain alert. Good sources of protein for breakfast and midday pick-ups are yogurt, cottage cheese, nuts and tofu, as well as obvious sources, such as meat, milk, eggs and cheese.

Because the B-complex vitamins are chemically related and may perform similar functions in the brain, a lack of one B vitamin adversely affects optimal absorption and utilization of the others.

- **Thiamine:** Lowered levels of vitamin B1 causes short-term memory problems, lack of coordination, and feelings of lassitude. Thiamine is needed to produce and use acetylcholine, one of the brain's major chemical messengers.

- **Niacin:** A lack of vitamin B3 can cause depression, emotional instability and loss of recent memory.

- **Pyridoxine:** Vitamin B6 is essential in the synthesis of GABA, a neurotransmitter that acts as a natural tranquilizer. Vitamin B6 is involved in the production of dopamine and serotonin. Pyridoxine deficiency is associated with depression.

- **Cobalimin:** Vitamin B12 deficiencies are linked with poor memory, inability to concentrate and decreased abstract thinking skills, as well as more severe mental effects such as psychosis, severe memory loss, and confusion. A deficiency can cause brain and spinal cord degeneration, and is linked with impaired production of acetylcholine.

- **Folic Acid:** Folic acid is found in leafy greens. A deficiency causes irritability and forgetfulness. With vitamin B12, folic acid plays a large role in the brain's production of acetylcholine.

- **Lecithin and Choline:** Other B-complex nutrients that maintain and enhance the brain's ability to reason, learn and remember are lecithin and choline. Laboratory experiments showed that animals given choline performed as well as younger animals on mental tests. Other tests have shown choline's ability to improve memory and maximize brain function. In an aging brain, cell membranes become rigid with fatty deposits and lose the ability to absorb and release brain chemicals and relay messages. This results in memory loss and confused thinking. Cells also lose dendritic spines, electrical-impulse carrying receptors necessary for information processing. A diet rich in lecithin and choline can retard age symptoms by stopping or delaying membrane hardening and dendritic spine loss. Choline also contributes to optimal brain performance by increasing the rate of the brain's metabolism. It maintains the structural integrity of the synapses, which are the points of communication between brain cells, and it is the substance from which the brain makes acetylcholine, a memory function neurotransmitter. Brain foods, such as fish, liver and eggs, supply lecithin and choline. Other good sources of lecithin and choline are cabbage, cauliflower and soybeans.

— ANTIOXIDANTS —

• Antioxidants can help your brain retain its sharp edge. The brain has many fat-containing cells, which are particularly vulnerable to damage from free radicals. Antioxidants beta-carotene, vitamins C and E, zinc and selenium can guard against free-radical damage and prevent the premature aging of brain cells.

— NEUROTRANSMITTERS —

- **Tryptophan and Serotonin:** This amino acid helps the brain synthesize serotonin, a necessary neurotransmitter involved in sleep, mental stability, coping with anxiety and regulating pain.

BE A HOT HEAD

Your internal temperature corresponds to your mental alertness—the warmer you are, the sharper your mind. The body is regulated by an internal clock attuned to the daily pattern of darkness and light, which affects your heart and respiration rate, blood pressure and body temperature. Generally, body temperatures are highest in the late afternoon and lowest before dawn, although individual temperature peaks can vary.

Monitor your temperature over a period of four or five days to discover your own body heat pattern. Use an oral thermometer and take your temperature every hour during the waking day. Avoid having a drink for 30 minutes before taking a measurement as the temperature of the drink will affect the thermometer. You'll see a pattern of peaks and dips corresponding to your mental performance pattern. Once you identify your personal peak times, you can take full advantage of them.

— MINERALS —

Trace minerals are essential for powerful brain function.

- **Zinc:** Adequate amounts of this mineral are essential for lasting brain health. Zinc is neces-

sary for the growth, development and functioning of the brain. It affects neurotransmitters,
brain wave patterns, the brain's physical struc-
tures, even the thinking process. Zinc deficiency includes symptoms of mental lethargy
and apathy.

- **Iron:** Iron-poor blood impairs the production
  and function of hemoglobin, an oxygen-trans-
  porting protein giving the blood its rich red
  color. Iron is heavily concentrated in the reticu-
  lar activating system, which turns the brain on
  and maintains alertness. Iron is an important
  component of several neurotransmitters, including serotonin, dopamine and noradrenaline. High
  levels of iron can improve verbal fluency, sus-
  tain attention and increase vigor. At high risk
  for low iron levels are women between 18 and
  44; dieters and the elderly, who eat less food;
  and vegetarians, since iron is most plentiful in
  meats and fish. If you are vegetarian, food
  sources rich in iron include blackstrap molasses,
  lima beans, soybeans, sunflower seeds, spinach,
  and broccoli. Iron absorption can be blocked by
  antacids, tea, phosphate additives in food and
  beverages, and the preservative EDTA, as well
  as some medications. Eating foods rich in vitamin C assists in optimal iron absorption.

- **Magnesium, Copper, Iodine and Manganese:**
  These are critical brain-nutrient minerals. They
  can affect brain functioning and mood, boost
  mental alertness, improve memory, reduce nervous anxiety and help keep you mentally stable.
  Magnesium functions as a natural tranquilizer;

a lack of magnesium results in extreme nervousness and irritability. Magnesium functions synergistically with the B vitamins to nourish the nerves and brain, and aids in the transmission of neural messages. Good sources of these minerals include dried beans, peas, shrimp, oysters and most seafood, onions, whole grains, leafy green vegetables, prunes, seeds, nuts, and fruits.

IONIZING THE BRAIN

Brain efficiency is affected by the ratio of positive to negative ions in the air. People feel better and are more productive when exposed to higher levels of negative ions. This causes lower levels of serotonin in the brain, thus relieving depression and sleepiness. If you spend much time in an enclosed office environment or a car, consider adding more negative ions to your environment with an ion generator.

— HEAVY METALS —

The heavy metals we're discussing here are not to be confused with rock music. Heavy metals—aluminum, mercury, lead and cadmium—are toxic to the brain at certain levels. Lead poisoning can cause mental sluggishness, and in high doses, mental retardation. Cadmium diminishes mental function and can lead to memory loss. Aluminum has been implicated in the development of Alzheimer's disease, which surfaces later in life. These toxic minerals have a cumulative effect, and the symptoms may not appear for years.

Be aware of possible exposure to toxic levels. You may be at risk if:

- You live in an area with high levels of environmental pollution, such as smog or smoke.

- You live near a freeway or airport. Engine exhausts contaminate the area with dangerously high levels of lead.

NOISE POLLUTION

Loud, noisy surroundings stress not only the body but the mind. Loud noise acts as a danger signal, causing the body to release adrenaline into the bloodstream, elevating blood pressure, increasing breathing and heart rate and affecting attention, memory and recall. If you can't put a stop to the noise, invest in some earplugs or headphones that will block the sound.

Another solution is to mask the offending sound with white noise, which is a bland, background sound similar to the radio hiss. A popular way to deal with distracting background noise is to listen to soothing new age music or environmental tapes.

- You cook in aluminum pots or with aluminum foil. Acidic foods, such as tomato juice, lemonade, vinegar, and orange juice, will draw the aluminum into them.

- You use an anti-perspirant containing aluminum. Over a period of time, you may be absorbing excess aluminum through the skin.

- You regularly take over-the-counter antacid remedies. One of the main ingredients in them is aluminum. Over a period of time, you could be getting too much aluminum. Avoid this by limiting your use of such remedies.

- You have silver fillings in your teeth. Silver fillings can release toxic metals into the body.

- You eat from ceramic bowls and dishes with lead glazes, which can leach into acidic foods.

Zinc, manganese and magnesium can reduce blood aluminum levels. Other nutritional supplements to detoxify your body of these toxic substances are glutathione, cysteine, vitamin C and selenium. These supplements will help your body flush out the heavy metal residue.

Using The Little Grey Cells

If there were a poster boy for bad habits, it would have to be Winston Churchill. Here was a man who defied medical advice. He puffed on noxious cigars, ate a very unhealthy diet, was overweight and didn't exercise much, and savored his Scotch regularly. In short, he lived an extremely unhealthy lifestyle. Common wisdom would indicate that his bad habits should have killed him at an early age, but he lived to the ripe age of ninety. He did one thing whose life-enhancing qualities seem to have outweighed all his bad habits—he kept his brain constantly active and challenged, and lived a productive, creative life.

Intense, concentrated mental activity, coupled with a

curiosity about the world around you, brings about an increased interaction with the process of life, which seems to slow down the aging process.

BRAIN ALLERGIES

Most people think of allergies as skin rashes and runny noses, but brain allergies can be responsible for mental fatigue, tension, dizziness, confusion, memory loss, and poor concentration.

One person in three is allergic to something in their environment, and anything can trigger an allergic reaction. Hypersensitivity tends to be genetic—are members of your family allergy prone? Do you suffer from puffy, baggy eyes or dark circles under the eyes; red, puffy ear lobes; scaly red patches on the cheeks; continual nasal drip? Do you display Jekyll & Hyde personality changes?

Any of these symptoms could indicate allergy syndrome. If so, the next step is to identify the substance responsible. Once identified, remove it from your environment or take steps to adapt to it.

This increased mental activity stimulates the little grey brain cells, the neurons. Each neuron has its own cell body and nucleus, as well as small filaments or branches which are vital to brain function. These filaments, called dendrites, number among the thousands. Their function is to provide connection to other brain cells. There are more than one trillion nerve cells in our brain, each with thousands of dendrites. Nerve impulses travel over the dendrites, carrying information to and from the brain. These connections are called synapses. The communication through these connections is called "thinking."

PLAIN OLD HORSE SENSE

Doctors propose a simple strategy to assist your memory that is called "intellectual self-management." This is a fancy title for common sense. Examples:

- If the weather forecast is for rain, immediately hook your umbrella over the front door knob. When you leave, you won't forget it.

- Keep a notepad or tape recorder at your bedside to enable you to capture creative ideas that spring into your head at night.

- Maximize your intellectual output by recording ideas, names and numbers in a pocket notebook; this allows for easy retrieval.

- Keeping your sentences short and to the point will enable you to avoid losing your train of thought in a conversation.

- Make an outline when writing to help prevent repetition and inconsistency.

— COGNITIVE TRAINING—

Cognitive training is not only the best way to maximize your biological potential by keeping your brain sharp, but it can even reverse physiological deterioration that may have already started in the brain. Too many of us equate mental exercise with boring, rote lessons, but it can be enjoyable and fun. Trying something absolutely new just

TO SLEEP, PERCHANCE TO IMPROVE THE MIND

Shakespeare knew the value of a good night's sleep. Sound sleep is a key factor in increasing brain performance. During sleep, the brain goes through a series of psychological processes restoring both body and mind. Chronic loss of sleep or otherwise disturbed sleep patterns affects mental clarity, decision making and attentiveness.

- A program of regular exercise can help you sleep better at night and may even reduce the amount of sleep you need, but avoid vigorous exercise just before bed as it overstimulates the body.

- Practice stress-releasing behaviors during the day: meditation, recreational reading or other relaxing mental outlets you enjoy.

- If you suffer from insomnia, avoid afternoon or early evening naps.

- Replace the after-dinner cup of coffee or caffeinated soda with decaffeinated coffee, soda, or herbal tea. Cut back or cut out the number of drinks you have before bedtime, since alcohol upsets rhythmic sleep patterns.

- Carbohydrates, starchy or sweet foods eaten at the evening meal will produce more serotonin, leading to a relaxed, drowsy feeling for a good night's sleep.

- Establish and maintain a regular bedtime routine— studies show that animals whose sleep schedule is frequently shifted have a 25% shorter lifespan.

for the fun of it is a wonderful exercise for your brain. A young child at play is actually exercising his mind constantly while he is learning new things and stimulating the mental neurons and synapses. The brain's adaptability and diversity has been called the prime identifying characteristic of our being.

The brain is elastic; it will continue to grow as long as it is challenged and stimulated. Like other parts of the body, if the brain is not stimulated, it atrophies. Constantly learning new things or doing things in a new, creative way causes organic changes in the brain—the nerve connections grow more complex, with more synapses. The greater the exposure to an environment that makes you use your brain, the more efficient and sharper your mind will become.

Scientists report brain growth even in very old rats when their environments were enriched with objects the rats could explore, and that were periodically exchanged for new objects. This was true even for rats who had lived in unenriched environments most of their lives before being transferred to more stimulating conditions. Their brains showed a higher content of noradrenaline, a strong nerve stimulant, and they more closely resembled the brains of healthy younger animals by showing increased thickness in the outer layers of the cerebral cortex, which represent an increase in dendrites, and they exhibited increased learning skills. This environmental enrichment required only a few days of stimulation in the young rats to show marked differences.

Good activities to keep your mind limber and agile include:

- **Language Abilities:** Learn a new one, or brush up on the language you are fluent in. Take a course at a community college or adult-education center. Challenge yourself—pick up one of the many preparation books available for the SAT or other standardized scholastic tests.

- **Visualization and Imagination:** Reading is particularly useful in sharpening these skills.

- **Reasoning:** Card games are particularly helpful to train reasoning and increase retention.

- **Problem-Solving:** Games such as puzzles, Scrabble, word jumbles, acrostics and interactive computer games stimulate the brain and give it needed exercise.

- **Spatial Skills:** Hobbies that focus your spatial skills by manipulating three-dimensional objects include model-building, sculpting, and painting. Take tests designed to sharpen specific skills of spatial orientation and inductive reasoning.

- **Concentration:** Improve your powers of concentration. Though absent-mindedness is frequently portrayed as being endearing and lovable, it can also be hazardous. Meditation and biofeedback are especially useful tools in learning to concentrate. Don't worry about things you have no control over, and don't burden your mind with thoughts that have no relevance to the situation at hand. How can the mind focus on the activities at hand? Look upon each day as a compartment of time and concentrate on what needs to be done during that time, neither looking backward to what might have been done nor forward to what is yet to be done. You can break the day into hourly compartments. This will help you calmly and methodically concentrate your mind intently, directing your thoughts and efforts on the business at hand.

- **Organization:** Cluttered surroundings can lead to a cluttered mind, in turn decreasing productivity and efficiency. Learn to organize your surroundings. If you are at a loss where to begin, many community colleges offer courses in organizing skills.

SLEEP PATTERNS

An interesting study by the Sleep Center of Boston State Hospital reports that those who sleep less tend to be efficient, ambitious, and highly programmed individuals. Those who sleep a lot tend to be more neurotic and nonconformist.

- **Lateral Thinking:** This consists of learning to look at things differently. Wide-focus your attention rather than narrowing it to small details, and don't be afraid to speculate. If you're having a problem that's hard to verbalize, switch to visual or abstract thinking mode. The ability to verbalize is centered in the left brain while visualization is located in the right brain. Be receptive and uncritical of the thoughts and ideas springing up in your mind.

- **Developing Creativity:** Creativity is not an

inborn trait. Like memory or concentration, it is a mental capacity that can be developed. The main elements are inspiration and perseverance. Inspiration isn't a thunderbolt from the blue; each of us has moments of inspiration throughout the day. What turns inspiration into creativity is perseverance. Creativity requires time, patience, concentration, and hard work. To stimulate creativity, practice the following steps: First, unfocus your thoughts and don't worry about being logical. Next, take a few minutes to perform a complete body/mind relaxation, then follow with at least 20 to 30 minutes of conscious imagery. Creativity involves exploring the unknown, combining thoughts and ideas in new ways. The creative process is the expression of people who are actualizing themselves.

Anything that enhances your adaptability to change can be included in an effective program of mental rejuvenation. Building these kinds of mental exercises into your life on a regular basis will make the physical changes in your brain's structure that reduce your effective mental age.

— MEMORY —

There are two kinds of memory: short term and long term. Short-term memory is comparable to the "in" basket on an office desk, while long-term memory is the file cabinet. Everything that comes into the brain (the office) goes through the in-basket (short-term memory) for review, but not everything gets filed in the filing cabinet (long-term memory).

THE ABSENT-MINDED PROFESSOR

Forgetfulness is not necessarily an early indication of senility. Albert Einstein is universally recognized as one of the most creative people who ever lived and a bona fide genius.

One evening, while working at Princeton University, he was forced to call the switchboard to find out where he lived. He had forgotten. He told the switchboard operator that he would have called home, but the number was unlisted and he couldn't remember that, either.

As children in school, we were taught to memorize things, but many of us never moved the memory into permanent storage. We tend to remember most easily what we want to remember. When we have an interest in something, remembering is effortless. The memory chain involves need or interest, attention, and organization. Memories tend to stick better when they are associated with an emotion, a sensory impression or a vivid experience. When any of these elements is lacking, we tend to forget.

Learn to use memory magnifiers. A good memory is one of the most impressive aspects of clear mental functioning, and loss of memory is the first sign associated with aging mental faculties. The ability to remember is nothing more than being able to register something, retain the memory, and retrieve it later. Memory can be assisted by associating the item we want to remember with a cue—a rhyme, word, place, or object. The more you practice remembering, the easier it will become. It is a skill that needs to be used daily.

There are three methods of improving the memory:

1) **Mechanical methods**, such as intensive study and repetition. This is the method most commonly used in schoolrooms, enabling children to learn the alphabet.

2) **Judicious methods,** which are based on logic, classification and analysis.

3) **Ingenious methods,** such as those listed below.

- **Mnemonics and Acronyms:** These are techniques of creating a word or sentence whose letters stand for one of the words you want to recall. "My Very Elegant Mother Just Served Us Nine Pizzas" is an easy way to remember the planets in our solar system in their correct order. "Every Good Boy Does Fine" represents the treble clef musical staff E, G, B, D, F. Recall the names of the five Great Lakes— Huron, Ontario, Michigan, Erie, and Superior—by thinking of the word "homes." You can remember anything with this technique.

- **Rhyme Association:** Match whatever you want to recall with a rhyming word—a rhyme is to the ear what a picture is to the eye. These rhymes about history, the calendar and spelling are good examples: "In fourteen hundred and ninety-two, Columbus sailed the ocean blue." "Thirty days hath September, April, June, and November, (etc.)" and "I before E except after C, or when sounded as A as in neighbor and weigh."

- **Visual Association:** Associate the item you want to remember with a visual cue. This works

JOG YOUR MEMORY

Studies measuring mental function after a 10-week program of jogging, calisthenics and other physical recreation showed significant improvements in intelligence, speed of performance, learning, and brain function, as well as decreased depression and lowered anxiety. Memory, attention span and motivation are also positively affected by exercise. A 20-30 minute aerobic workout produces an almost instantaneous mental lift as well. Why? It oxygenates the bloodstream, enabling the body to better transport oxygen to all its organs.

Like other organs, the brain relies on the blood to provide oxygen and nutrients while carrying away carbon dioxide and other waste products. The brain uses oxygen to oxidize glucose in the production of electrical energy, speeding up the nerve impulses between brain cells. Shallow breathing and clogged arteries leave the brain gasping for air. Build a better brain while improving your physique.

A number of studies show that the mental reaction times of athletes are faster than those of nonathletes. Exercise increases the amount of the stimulating neurotransmitter, noradrenaline, in the brain. When people with low fitness levels begin physical training, their reaction times improve.

If you dislike strenuous physical exertion, take heart. Even moderate physical activity is accompanied by positive electrical and chemical changes in the brain, a strengthening of the dominant brain-wave frequency, and increased levels of neurotransmitters dopamine and noradrenaline, as well as endorphins, the body's natural opiates.

especially well with names, but be careful if you use silly images to remember someone's name. You don't want to alienate them by laughing every time you use their name.

- **Grouping:** It's helpful to break long strings of information into groups consisting of no more than five pieces of information. Think of your social security number, for example. It's only nine numbers long, yet most of us memorized it by breaking it into three groups of numbers.

- **Location Association:** To recall a list of things, envision an area you are familiar with, then locate each item on the list in this familiar landscape. To remember the list, simply take a mental tour through the area.

SMOKE GETS IN YOUR BRAIN

Researchers measuring the verbal recall performance of smokers discovered that the nicotine in cigarette smoke interferes with short-term memory. One study compared 37 smokers with 37 nonsmokers. Subjects were tested on the recall of the names of 12 people. Nonsmokers correctly recalled an average of 9 names out of 12 (75 percent) while smokers averaging a pack a day could only remember 6 names (50 percent).

Other factors that negatively influence memory may be lurking in your medicine chest. Prescription drugs such as blockers and calcium-channel blockers can cause brain drain by slowing your heart rate, thus slowing the oxygen supply to the brain. Certain nonsteroidal anti-inflammatory drugs can impair blood flow in some people, increasing the risk of memory loss, inability to concentrate and confusion. If you suspect that any prescription drug is causing memory problems, discuss the problem with your physician **before** making any decisions to discontinue the medication.

While not extremely common, even over-the-counter medications can cause mental impairment. Antihistamines impair the function of cholinergic neurons, brain chemicals that are used in thought processes, leading to decreased ability to concentrate and grogginess. Other potentially mind-dulling medications: antidiarrheal agents containing paregoric can cause drowsiness; analgesics such as ibuprofen can cause drowsiness or dizziness; cough suppressants containing codeine, dextromethorphan or diphenhydramine can have sedative effects; anti-nausea drugs containing meclizine or dimenhydrinate can have sedative effects; and sleeping aids containing antihistamines—after you wake up, the antihistamines can remain active for up to six hours, which means you'll still be feeling drowsy.

Stress

De-stressing is a popular pastime in our modern culture. People are constantly looking for effective ways to relieve themselves of stress. People with strong psychological coping skills have been found to have more powerful immune systems, and higher levels of killer immune cells than people with poor coping skills. These people are said to have self-healing personalities.

POSTURE

Since mankind first stood erect, every mother's favorite phrase has echoed in our ears. When you stand up straight, with your head back and chin tucked in, you'll not only look and feel better, you'll think better too. Hunched-over posture pinches arteries connecting the spinal column to the brain, decreasing blood flow to the brain and resulting in fuzzy thinking and forgetfulness. Eventually, these disturbances cause an accumulation of fatty deposits that can lead to transient ischemic attacks—brief blackouts similar to stroke symptoms. You can prevent this by properly aligning your body.

Physical stress causes premature aging by switching on a primitive "fight or flight" reaction that causes an outpouring of hormones. Adrenaline rushes into the blood stream, and turns off the thymus gland, a key component of the immune system. Blood pressure rises, and heart rate increases. The body reacts by shutting down activity in the digestive tract; blood shifts from the abdominal organs to those essential to muscular exertion and activity; increased heart muscle contractions occur; extra red blood cells are discharged from the spleen into the bloodstream to carry more oxygen to the muscles; deeper breathing and dilation of the lung's bronchial tubes occur, and blood sugar flows out of the liver to answer the increased energy demands. Mental and physical stress stimulate the hypothalamus.

SEEING THE LIGHT

Light has a definite biobehavioral effect on humans by stimulating the pineal gland, which regulates melatonin, a blood hormone. Stimulation of the pineal gland relieves depression and activates other important biochemical events in our bodies involved in endocrine control, timing of our biological clocks, entrainment of circadian rhythms, immunologic responsiveness, sexual growth and development, regulation of stress and fatigue, control of viral infection, and dampening functional disorders of the nervous system. If we are to feel energetic and to perform at our best, our bodies need to be exposed to full-spectrum light.

Mood and performance suffer when light levels are irregular or too little. People who work in urban glass-and-concrete caves with artificial lighting, those living in the far north, or city-dwellers surrounded by heavy smog or endlessly overcast days need to make special efforts to get more exposure to natural, full-spectrum light, especially during winter months when days are shorter.

Timing of light exposure is also important. People whose schedules cause them to miss dawn or dusk or both experience artifically shortened daylight periods. Without the biological cues which regulate their internal clocks, eating and sleeping patterns are thrown off, as well as hormonal and neurotransmitter release in the brain.

When people are in stressful situations for prolonged periods of time, these reactions remain switched on, leading to complete exhaustion of the autonomic nervous system and lowering immunological response to disease. The body is seriously compromised in its ability to fight off infection and disease.

Mental stress is the brain's number one enemy. It can produce anxiety and worry, and narrow your focus of attention so important cues and perceptions are missed. Your brain performs best when you are in a calm relaxed state of mind. Though your brain can occasionally perform awe-inspiring feats while under tremendous pressure, continuing tension, turmoil and anxiety clutter your mind, decreasing thinking ability.

The effects of stress on the body are very real, yet stress is a subjective phenomenon. What may seem very stressful to one individual might cause another person to shrug and proceed to forget about it. How a situation is perceived plays a larger part in your responses than the actuality of that situation. When you interpret a situation and form an assumption, that assumption continues to operate without your conscious knowledge.

Emotional factors interfering with mind-body interaction are fear, anger and guilt. All other negative feelings are directly related to these three. Fear and anger evolved from basic survival instincts, modified by social expectations, while guilt is man-made, the result of judgments and evaluations based on social customs, expectations and values. Learn to detach from these negative emotions and allow them to flow past without affecting you.

A certain amount of stress is the price everyone pays for living. Most of life's events can't be avoided and must be lived through. How do you handle it? Ask yourself whether you have any control over the situation; if the answer is 'no,' recognize that whatever is happening is a random coincidental event that has nothing to do with you. Try not to personalize the event. Be reasonably vigilant and accept that a certain amount of risk is part of being alive. Put the events in perspective by challenging irrational beliefs. Diminish your reaction to what you read or hear by one-half. We need to be alert as to when stress becomes distress and break the cycle before it gets the upper hand. What we don't want is a cycle of constant distress.

It may seem difficult to deliberately force yourself not to worry, but worry is directly related to physical tension. Ease the physical tension and your mind will follow. Soothing music, progressive relaxation training, deep breathing, meditation, and yoga are useful to achieve a calm emotional state and reduce mental clutter.

BE A CRYBABY

When you feel sad, go ahead and cry. It's not only okay to express your emotions, but you may lower your risk of developing serious disease by not suppressing your feelings.

Tears are the byproduct of the body's waste-removal system. Tears that are shed in grief or sorrow carry off stress-related chemicals. People who suppress their emotions and condition themselves not to cry are more susceptible to stress-related diseases, such as ulcers, hardening of the arteries and heart attacks.

— YOGA —

Yoga benefits the mind as well as the body. The process of stretching, tensing and flexing the muscles in these age-old postures will balance your entire being. Following are some invigorating warm-ups followed by some basic yoga postures. Never strain to accomplish a position; with each repetition, you'll get better. As you get better, the postures will become automatic. After you have mastered these positions, you may wish to further your benefits by enrolling in a yoga class.

INVIGORATING WARM-UPS

Chest Expander—A Stretching Warm-Up

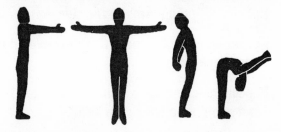

- Stand up straight, arms extended forward and touch palms.

- Extend arms slowly to the side. Then clasp hands behind back, arms straight down.

- Inhale deeply, pulling shoulders back.

- Holding the breath, slowly bend forward and raise your arms high over your head.

- Exhale. Slowly return to the original position.

- Repeat once.

The Pulley—A Tensing Warm-Up

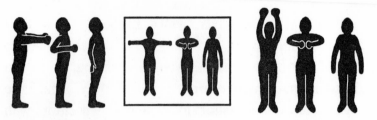

- Inhale and extend arms in front of the body at shoulder level.

- Continue holding the breath and make a fist, palms upward. Tense the upper part of your body. As though pulling a heavy weight, slowly move fists toward chest.

- Exhale, dropping arms to the side.

- Repeat the exercise, only this time extend your arms to the sides.

- Repeat the exercise, and this time extend your arms straight up over your head.

Rock 'n Rolls—A Flexing Warm-Up

- Beginners: Lie on your back. Slowly raise your knees and grasp your hands behind upper legs with fingers interlocking. Gently rock backward and forward on the spine. Don't roll too far when you first attempt this warm-up; repetition will allow you to rock further with time.

- Advanced: Sitting on the floor, cross your legs and grasp the right toe with your left hand and the left toe with your right hand. Without raising your buttocks, lower your head to the floor. Keep feet flat on the floor. Maintaining the grip on your toes, rock all the way back onto your shoulders until your hands and toes touch the floor over your head. Hold briefly, then return to beginning position. Repeat two or three times until your body feels invigorated.

The Fountain Twist—A Balancing Warm-Up

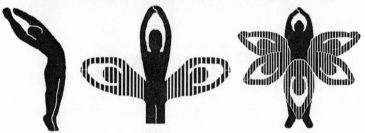

- Inhale deeply. Stretch your whole body upward, rising up on the balls of your feet and stretching your arms as high as possible over your head.

- Continue to stretch and hold, pulling up all along your spine.

- Exhale and relax.

- Inhale and again stretch body upward, rising up on the balls of your feet, and stretching your arms over your head. This time, hook your thumbs together.

- Holding your breath, bend to the right as far as you can. Return up right, then bend as far to the left as you can.

- Exhale and relax.

- Inhale. Stretch your body, then bend forward, rotating the upper part of your body in a full circle. Feel your waist stretching as you do this exercise.

- Return to upright position, exhale and relax.

- Repeat forward bend, circling in the other direction.

BASIC YOGA POSITIONS
The Plough

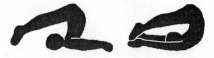

- Lie flat on your back, arms extended at your side. Raise your legs slowly while inhaling. Keep your palms flat against the floor.

- Without bouncing or bending your knees, continue to raise your hips and back slowly. Bring the legs all the way over your head until your toes touch the floor behind you.

- Swing arms back and grab your toes.

- Breathing slowly through your nose, press your chin against your chest. Hold for two minutes, or as long as you can at first.

- Then bring legs slowly back to the floor.

- Straighten your arms and return slowly to a sitting position.

Forward Bend (Sitting)

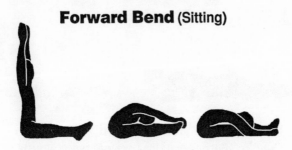

- This is a deceptively simple exercise. In a sitting position, raise your arms high over your head, stretching the spine upward. Inhale deeply.

- Exhale. Slowly lean forward (don't bounce) and grab your toes without bending your knees.

- Hold for as long as is comfortable, then return to sitting position.

Half Locust

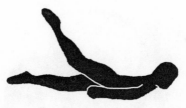

- Lie face down, hands by your sides, palms up.

- Inhale. Raise your right leg, keeping the knee straight. Do not move the other leg. Stretch the leg up as far as possible.

- Hold for a count of ten.

- Release the breath and lower your leg. Repeat with other leg.

- Alternate legs three more times.

The Cobra

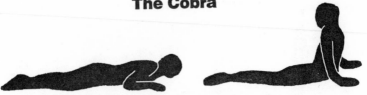

- Lie flat on the stomach. Fold your arms at the sides so that your palms are pressing against the floor at shoulder level, fingers outstretched.

- Slowly raise your head, neck and upper back as far as possible. Your lower body should remain flat on the floor, from your belly-button down. Hold for 15 to 30 seconds.

- Return to floor.

Triangle Posture

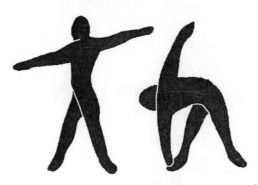

- Stand erect, feet two feet apart, and extend your arms straight out from the body.

- Twist your trunk from the waist, turning as far around as possible.

- Bending, touch one hand to opposite foot, keeping the other arm aligned perpendicular to body.

- Hold the stretch for a few seconds, then return to standing position and repeat with other side.

Leg Split

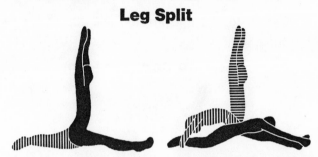

- From a kneeling position, lift your left leg and extend it forward while the right leg is stretching back to form a split.

- Raise hands over head, stretching the spine.

- Inhale, then stretch backward so your spine forms an arc. Hold briefly, exhale and return to original position.

- Repeat on other side.

Deep Lunge

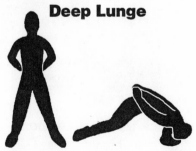

- Stand erect, feet two feet apart, and clasp your hands behind your back.

- Slowly flex your right knee and bend trunk, reaching for your toes.

- Try to touch forehead to toes and hold for 20 to 30 seconds.

- Return to starting position and repeat for the other side.

Forward Bend (Standing)

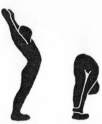

- Stand straight. Inhale and raise your arms over your head as high as you can.

- Bend slowly down while exhaling, pressing your face into your knees while touching your toes. Your legs should remain straight. Hold for several seconds.

- Inhale; straighten up. Repeat two or three times.

Resting Pose

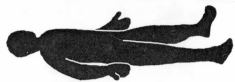

- This pose finishes all yoga sessions. Lie on your back, arms straight along your sides, palms up.

- Close your eyes and relax your body, one part at a time, from toes to head. Breathe in slowly and deeply from the diaphragm while relaxing body parts.

—MEDITATION—

There is a large body of scientific research showing that meditation is more effective in the alleviation of anxiety than therapy. In a recent, large-scale "meta-analysis" (a statistical technique designed to compare research across a variety of studies), meditators have been shown to be significantly more self-actualized than psychotherapy patients. When scientifically compared to other self-growth techniques, meditation has more physiological impact than standard biofeedback techniques, is more effective than waking imagery techniques and promotes significantly more body relaxation than simple eyes-closed rest.

The following meditation is a simple one that will foster inner-connectedness, leading to a sense of balance and integration with the world around you.

The Tree of Life

In this meditation, we will attune ourselves with the stream of energy that connects us with the Universe. This empowering exercise will bring this stream of energy into your awareness. This awareness will unify and focus the power and energies of your conscious and your subconscious mind, and enable you to manifest the Universal energy in your daily life.

Keep both feet flat on the floor. Close your eyes, take a deep breath and relax. Feel your body relaxing ... your hands and feet are now relaxing ... feel the relaxing power moving up your legs and arms ... and into your chest, your back, and your stomach ... you are now relaxed and at ease.

Focus on your breath coming into your body and going

out. As you inhale, you breathe in peace ... as you exhale, you breathe out tensions ... breathe in relaxation, breathe out anxiety ... breathe in light, breathe out darkness.

Now visualize a majestic tree growing from inside you. Sense yourself becoming one with the tree. Your body is the trunk of this glorious tree. Feel the branches and leaves growing out of your torso, and as you do, reach as far toward the sky overhead as is comfortable. The branches not only catch the rays of the sun; they also catch the light and power of the energy that is constantly moving throughout eternity. That light and power enters through the leaves and moves down into you, filling your being with its majesty and purpose.

The energy moves through you, then leaves through the soles of your feet, which are the tree's roots. Direct your awareness into your feet. Feel the energy in your feet and move it down into the roots that grow out of your feet and on into the ground, down deeply into the earth itself ... as deeply into the earth as you feel comfortable.

What do your roots look like? Some of the roots might be thin, others might be thicker or sturdier. Feel these roots interlocking and working through the earth. Feel the deep, dark places of your being in your roots, and allow yourself to sense the energy that pulses through them, compacted deeply in your roots. Remove any blocks or knots in the roots that keep the Divine energy from being available in your life and allow it to begin to flow freely through you.

Now visualize this energy going deeper still, cupping itself around and circling the ball of fire in the center of the earth. See it moving back up, passing through your root system and rushing through the former blocks and kinks and flowing up through your body. Feel it sweep through the branches and leaves and out into the sky. You are the conductor for this divine power.

Feel the vertical line of energy flowing through your body, centering you with the heaven above and the earth below, moving up through you and expressing itself in the upward reach of your branches. Let the top of the tree now reach as high as you want. Experience how it feels to be centered and in alignment with the Universe.

Maintain the awareness of the light and power of your tree as much as possible throughout the activities of your day. When this happens, your spirit embraces the Divine. Say quietly to yourself: I dedicate my life to the loving expression of the power within me. Through dedication, I unfold naturally to the highest potential of my being.

LOOK YOUNGER WITH
— AN ATTITUDE ADJUSTMENT—

There is a youth elixir that is absolutely, positively guaranteed to make you look at least five to ten years younger. Better than that, it will make you ageless. But you can't buy this elixir—you have to make it yourself. It's joy. It's happiness. It's contentment. Being happy with yourself despite circumstances or surroundings. At any age, a cheerful, happy face is more attractive and looks younger than one with a scowl or a droopy look. Cheerful people are more enjoyable to be around because their enthusiasm and joy for life attract people to them.

You can develop this positive, life-enhancing, beautifying quality through an attitude adjustment—toward others, toward the world, and most importantly toward yourself.

Be less critical of others—resentment breeds illness. By resenting others, dwelling on perceived injuries and holding onto your anger, you'll be the one who gets sick, not them. Fear, depression, anger, and negative emotions are strong immune system depressors. Don't get upset and excited over every little thing that happens, especially when it does not affect you or is no concern of yours. Release the negative feeling and let it flow out of you; feel yourself becoming happier and more content.

THE HALF-EMPTY GLASS

The way you explain an event is a good indicator of your orientation toward life. Studies show that a pessimistic outlook is strongly linked to poor health.

- Poor problem-solving skills are linked with pessimism. Pessimism-related feelings of helplessness affect the immune function.

- Pessimism may lead to social withdrawal and isolation—behavior that is associated with illness.

- People with pessimistic outlooks are consistently sicker than their peers.

Negative thinking has a powerful impact on your potential for longevity, adversely affecting not only your brain's performance but your immune system as well. Yet we all fall into these habits periodically—overgeneralizing, jumping to conclusions, and indulging in "if only" and "I should have" thinking. All-or-nothing thinking can lead to anxiety, depression, guilt, perfectionism, anger, and feelings of inferiority. Learn to think in shades of grey, not black or white only.

There has been a lot of attention given to the subject of the effect of the mind on healing. Research findings show the importance of attitude adjustment on your health:

- Mental programming affects one's chances of getting and surviving many kinds of cancer, including lung, breast, cervical and skin cancers.

- Eternal optimist or pessimist—the personality programming you received as a child can affect the likelihood of developing cancer later in life.

- Optimists tend to be less bothered by physical symptoms than pessimists because optimists cope more effectively with problems and experience less stress-related symptoms.

- It is distressing and injurious to health to have responsibility but no sense of control. Feelings of helplessness, futility and lack of control can result in a lowered immune system response.

- Animals given control over their environment are able to fight off cancerous tumors better and live longer than animals with no control.

- Institutionalized people given choices and more control over their lives show dramatic improvements in overall health, even reversing bodily changes due to aging.

- Personality type may play a role in a person's susceptibility to diseases like asthma, peptic ulcers, arthritis, diabetes, multiple sclerosis, heart disease and cancer.

- Brain chemicals that regulate happiness, sex drive, mental functioning, sleep, depression, aggression, and all of our other brain functions, have been found to activate specific immune fighters such as scavenger cells, killer T-cells, antibody-producing cells, and immune boosters like interferon and interleukin-2.

- Prolonged grieving, stress, and depression have all been proven to lower your body's immunological fighter cells dramatically.

- Medical researchers discovered that patients who are programmed to expect a slow recovery after surgery exhibit more physical problems, and those who expect to leave the hospital quickly are much more likely to.

- By using mental-relaxation tools, people can lower blood pressure and reduce the frequency of heart-rhythm abnormalities.

- Psychologists have discovered that people with multiple personalities have dramatically different physical reactions with each persona. Reactions include tolerance to medications, eyesight and sensory acuity, allergies, right- or left-handedness, and neurological characteristics. Mental programming for each personality transforms the same individual into many measurably different biological "beings."

We all have the need to love and be loved. Studies show that the socially isolated—those unmarried, divorced or widowed people with few close friends and few social contacts—are three times more likely to die of a wide variety of diseases than people who enjoy happy, fulfilling social lives. Forming close personal ties to friends, family and community can safeguard your health. Developing deep, loving relationships takes work. Be selective—devote the most energy to the relationships that matter the most to you. Cultivate candor—tell people what you really feel. Honest communication is the key to all relationships. Work together—most rewarding relationships have shared elements. Overlook petty flaws—unrealistic expectations can destroy relationships. If you really want the relationship to grow, don't expect perfection. Share everything—the good as well as sad or bad things.

HUGGING STRESS AWAY

Hugging is healthy. The human touch not only soothes, it heals, resulting in lower levels of stress hormones and a higher ratio of helper/suppressor T-cells, an important balance in a healthy immune system. Studies show that even patients in deep comas display improved heart rate and brainwaves when their hands are held by doctors, nurses, or family members.

Your relationship with yourself is the most important relationship you will ever have. Self-image plays an important part in the state of your health. An injured or low self-image can allow you to accept a state of mental, physical or emotional imbalance as normal. Since you are the creator of your own self-image and are the only one capable of changing, you must ask for and receive your own permission to change, every step of the way.

Release the negative emotions of anger, fear and guilt. Forgive yourself as well as others in order to release the past. Learn to love yourself and believe that you deserve to be healthy. Use daily positive affirmations to program a healthy lifestyle for yourself, and express gratitude and thankfulness for that health in advance, for it will soon become your reality.

LAUGHTER IS THE BEST MEDICINE

If there were a pill that lowered blood pressure, improved digestion, gave you better muscle tension and elevated your mood, all at the same time, wouldn't you take it? You don't have to take a pill to experience those effects—all you have to do is laugh. It has all the positive physical effects mentioned above, which can positively affect your health by helping you maintain a balanced perspective. Laughter blocks feelings of apprehension and panic that can accompany serious illness. Laughing makes things seem less frightening and overwhelming. Have fun, watch funny movies or read funny books, but incorporate laughter into your life.

FACING FORWARD

*F*uture *Potentials*

While you've been reading this book, somewhere a scientist may have discovered a youth formula that will make everything else obsolete. Most likely, it will be a technique or tool based on a newly discovered principle of longevity or development of the practical aspects of an "old wive's tale." Read on to discover some future potentials for not only extending our lives, but our looks as well.

The Face of The Future

...

The following tidbits are what lies ahead of us—scientific breakthroughs and future potentials that may profoundly affect your life and looks.

✧ SUPER JUICE ✧

Home juicing appliances have become popular in the last few years, but food companies are developing a new super juice that may outperform nature. They call them "lifecycle juices" and base their findings on the life-enhancing compounds found in the piths and peels of citrus fruits—substances called bioflavonoids. They take these antioxidant compounds and add them to orange juice. The juices discourage not only cholesterol oxidation but work to prevent excessive blood cell clotting.

Other potentials for fortified juices include orange juice

with cancer-fighting compounds such as d-limonene, or one with a memory enhancer.

✧ *PEPPER, PLEASE* ✧

Scientists are studying the pain-relieving effects of a cream containing capsaicin, an ingredient in fiery-hot peppers. When applied to the knees of experimental subjects, the cream relieved symptoms of rheumatoid arthritis and osteoarthritis by inhibiting the release of a neurotransmitter that sends pain signals to the brain.

✧ *PERFECTLY PIGGY* ✧

Chronic shortages of human donor organs and the improved effectiveness of anti-rejection drugs have doctors scrambling to find substitutes for life-saving hearts, lungs, kidneys and livers. British scientists are inserting human protein genes into the fertilized eggs of pigs. When the organs are harvested, the genes will mark them as human organs to the immune system, making them more easily accepted by the body.

✧ *HANG IT IN YOUR EAR* ✧

The most recent device to surface in the war against smoking is a tiny appliance designed to be inserted in the outer ear. It works by sending a weak electrical pulse into the ear, stimulating the nerve that runs from the brain, behind the ear and into the abdomen. The nerve signals the brain to release endorphins and enkephalins, the body's natural painkillers, into the system. When the smoker feels the urge to light up, he is instructed to insert the device and switch it on. Within a few minutes, the craving for a cigarette should be gone.

✧ THE PRINCE OF FROGS ✧

The natural defenses of the dart poison frog, inhabitant of South American rain forests, contain an alkaloid called epibatidine that has painkilling properties 100 to 400 times more potent than morphine. It works by blocking receptors in the brain that process pain signals. Scientists are working on synthesizing the compound.

TRANSPLANTING ✧ BRAIN CELLS ✧

In a scenario that sounds like a science fiction movie, researchers are growing brain cells in the laboratory. Cells taken from patients undergoing brain surgery are placed in a petri dish and treated with growth factors. The cells not only grew, they thrived. Interconnections between the cells grew and the cells began producing essential brain chemicals called neurotransmitters.

✧ FILLING IN THE LINES ✧

Threading, a technique to erase wrinkles, inserts threads between the dermis and the subcutaneous fatty tissue. Non-inflammatory scar tissue forms around the threads, plumping up the skin by as much as 60 percent.

FAT-BURNING
✧ METABOLISM BOOSTERS ✧

Studies on obese patients placed on a low-fat, high-fiber diet showed that when a new class of drugs were used, the patients lost 54 percent more weight after four months than a control group on the same diet. The drugs are called thermogenic beta-3 agonists and they work by boosting the metabolism during the period of reduced food intake.

✧ TEA POWDER ✧

Japanese green tea has long been regarded as a longevity-enhancing drink, but the actual tea leaves themselves get left behind when the tea has been drunk.

To obtain the most good from the tea, the Japanese are grinding the tea into a fine powder and adding it to food. Research by Japanese scientists indicate that green tea helps reduce blood fats and cholesterol, as well as being an anti-carcinogen.

✧ SWEET TOOTH ✧

From the land down under, Australian scientists have isolated a milk protein called casein phosphopeptide that replaces calcium phosphate in decaying teeth. The protein, when added to soft drinks and candy, would safeguard the teeth against decay. One can't help but wonder what dentists will do?

NOT JUST FOR VAMPIRE
✧ PROTECTION ANYMORE ✧

Alliin, a precursor of allicin, the component scientists believe to be the active ingredient in garlic, lowered bad cholesterol levels by 11 percent in recent studies. The compound was distilled from garlic for use in the studies.

✧ ANTI-AGING APHRODISIAC ✧

Deprenyl, which is used to treat Parkinson's disease and depression, has demonstrated anti-aging and aphrodisiac effects in early studies.

✧ A VERY FISHY STORY ✧

Halfway through the lifecycle of the coho salmon, it suddenly grows new nerve cells throughout its brain. The neural pathways and neurotransmitters in the fish are very similar to humans, so the hormone that causes this regeneration could possibly work in humans as well. This could pave the way for new treatments that could repair damage from brain diseases like Parkinson's and Alzheimer's— age-related cell-degenerating diseases.

✧ REGENERATING ENZYMES ✧

Test-tube experiments with the enzyme phosphoglycerate kinase (PGK) are pointing the way to new treatments for treating the body's enzymes so they stay young forever. As enzymes age, they become flaccid and lose their ability to function. Researchers soaked old enzymes in a chemical solution that returned the enzymes to their original structure. PGK enzymes are vital to the healthy functioning of the heart, lungs and other internal organs, so rejuvenating these enzymes could slow down or reverse the internal aging process.

✧ SPRAYING FLU AWAY ✧

Australian researchers are testing a drug that may knock out the flu bug. Because the flu virus has shown an amazing ability to mutate, defeating attempts to kill it, vaccines have been notoriously ineffective in eliminating the virus. The new drug works by blocking neuraminidase, an enzyme that viruses piggy-back throughout the body. So far, the flu virus has not shown any mutation to develop resistance to the drug. Human tests of the drug are planned. The drug will be delivered into the body by an aerosol spray.

GREAT BARRIER
✧ SUNBLOCKER ✧

Australian scientists have discovered that algae growing in the coral that forms the Great Barrier Reef in Australia contains an amino acid that absorbs damaging ultraviolet radiation, including the dangerous UVB rays. This protects the coral from being destroyed by the sun's rays. They have synthesized a sunscreen from the amino acid, which is undergoing further testing.

About The Author

Sharon Boyd has been working in the publishing industry since 1976, and has written extensively for the New Age, self-help, and personal development markets. The associate editor of **Valley of the Sun Publishing** since 1982, she has worked with many well-known authors on their books. She lives in Agoura Hills, California, where she is tolerated by a 24-pound Maine Coon cat who does the "empty food bowl dance" at 4 a.m.

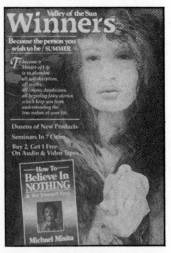

VIDEO HYPNOSIS® TAPES
Available Through Your Local Metaphysical Bookseller
Or Directly From Valley of the Sun Publishing

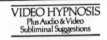
VIDEO HYPNOSIS
Plus Audio & Video
Subliminal Suggestions

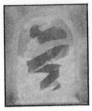

Increase
Self-Discipline

Generates An Eyes-Open Altered State of Conscious-
ness. Two Kinds of Hypnosis and Two Kinds of
Subliminal Programming Make This The Most
Powerful Self-Help Programming In The World.

Self-change doesn't get any easier or more powerful than this! With video, two extra dimensions of brain/mind technology are incorporated, resulting in four times the programming power: Visual hypnosis, as well as the verbal body relaxation and induction, and subliminal programming,which uses suggestions quickly flashed on the screen as well as embedded into the soothing background music. Thanks to this awareness of how the mind works, change no longer has to be difficult.This incredible four-way combination makes these videos the most powerful self-change tapes in the world. Thanks to this awareness of how the mind works, change no longer has to be difficult.

30 minutes/VHS only. . . . . $19.95 each

LOSE WEIGHT NOW
Examples of Suggestions
You control your weight. ■ Every day you become thinner. ■ You eat smaller portions at meals. ■ You quit all snacking. ■ You stick to your diet. ■ You live a healthy lifestyle. ■ A thin, healthy body is now your reality. ■ You now lose weight and fulfill your goals. .. VHS103—$19.95

REINVENT YOURSELF
Example of Suggestions
You now reinvent yourself. ■ You decide what you really want in life. ■ You make joyous choices that bring you peace. ■ You become committed to your values and goals. ■ You organize your time and energy to support your goals. ■ You enjoy communication. . . . . . VHS150—$19.95

PERFECT WEIGHT, PERFECT BODY
Example of Suggestions
You have the power and ability to attain the perfect weight and body. ■ You have the self-discipline to do what is required to attain the body you desire. ■ You live a healthy lifestyle and exercise daily. ■ You now attain your weight goals and the body you desire.. . . . . . VHS141—$19.95

INCREASE SELF-DISCIPLINE
Examples of Suggestions
You now have the self-discipline to accomplish your personal and professional goals. ■ You direct your time and energy to manifest your desires. ■ Every day in every way, you increase your self-discipline. ■ You do what you need to do and you stop doing what doesn't work.
. . . . VHS147—$19.95

RX17® AUDIO TAPES
Available Through Your Local Metaphysical Bookseller
Or Directly From Valley of the Sun Publishing

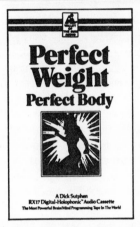

RX17® tapes incorporate state-of-the-art digital recording and the latest brain/mind technology to synchronize both halves of your brain. You are then receptive to new beliefs.

Side A: Alpha Level Programming: Descriptions of a tropical island beach at sunrise are integrated into a body relaxation; ocean waves roll in and out in digital 3-D sound. Subliminal "follow-response" technology lulls you into a soothing alpha level. Next, each tape delivers suggestions that use mind imprinting techniques to help create who and what you want to be!

Side B: Subliminal Programming: Contains 30 minutes of relaxing, digitally recorded stereo music. Each tape uses different music. Subliminal suggestions are synthesized and projected in the same chord and frequency as the music; only your subconscious mind hears. The suggestions are printed on the package. You may also use this side of the tape as **sleep programming.** Simply listen as you go to sleep; it is incredibly powerful.
.... **$12.50 each.**

A CALM & PEACEFUL MIND
Example of Suggestions
You are now at peace with yourself, the world and everyone in it. ■ Tranquility, harmony and a quietness of spirit permeate you. ■ You feel peaceful, balanced and harmonious.......... **RX103—$12.50**

PERFECT WEIGHT, PERFECT BODY
Example of Suggestions
You have the power and ability to attain the perfect weight and body. ■ You eat smaller portions at meals. ■ You live a healthy lifestyle. ■ You attain your weight goals and the body you desire.
.... **RX111—$12.50**

CREATIVE VISUALIZATION
Example of Suggestions
You visualize your desires with no indecisiveness at all. ■ What you visualize now manifests itself. ■ You hold a clear image and combine it with emotional desire.
.... **RX150—$12.50**

POSITIVE THINKING
Example of Suggestions
You see positive opportunities in everything you experience. ■ You are optimistic and enthusiastic. ■ You look forward to challenges. ■ You think positively. ■ You experience the joy and mentally detach from all negativity.
.... **RX148—$12.50**

SLEEP PROGRAMMING AUDIO TAPES
Available Through Your Local Metaphysical Bookseller
Or Directly From Valley of the Sun Publishing

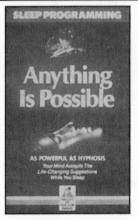

Sleep Programming is as powerful as hypnosis for programming your mind with life-changing suggestions! And all you have to do is listen to the tape as you go to sleep. The 30-minute (per side) program begins with **Dick Sutphen** directing a body relaxation. Behind his voice and soothing music is a brain/mind "follow response" sound that helps put you to sleep. You'll then hear from 750 to 1,000 words of paced, repeated suggestions interspersed with support phrases. The words fade away at the end of the tape telling you to sleep soundly through the night and awaken inspired to begin a new day.

.... **$10.98 each**

BE RELAXED AND STRESS FREE
Programming to develop the ability to detach from worldly pressures and retreat to a calm inner space. **Suggestion examples:** You peacefully accept the things you cannot change and change the things you can. A quietness of spirit permeates your body and mind. Much more. .... **1120—$10.98**

SELF-DISCIPLINE
You are encouraged to be self-disciplined and to accomplish your goals. **Suggestion examples:** You do what you need to do to accomplish your goals. You control your thoughts and thus your actions. You are assertive and feel good about yourself. You commit to your goals. .... **1105—$10.98**

ANYTHING IS POSSIBLE
Programming to convince you that anything is indeed possible. **Suggestion examples:** You do what you need to do. You do. You see positive opportunities in everything you experience, and you use them to create the life you want to live....... **1124—$10.98**

TOMORROW IS A NEW BEGINNING
Programs you to be confident and secure, to forgive yourself and others. **Suggestion examples:** Allow your Higher Self to guide you. The light of awareness now cleanses your mind of negativity. Your deepest desires are coming true. .... **1104—$10.98**

These titles may be purchased at your local New Age store, or you may order them directly from **Valley of the Sun Publishing**. VISA and MasterCard orders, call toll-free: 1-800-421-6603, or make checks payable to **Valley of the Sun Publishing**. Mail to:

Valley of the Sun Publishing
Box 38, Malibu, CA 90265